OPERATIVE HYSTEROSCOPY

OPERATIVE HYSTEROSCOPY

Hubert Guedj MD
Chief of Hysteroscopy
Faculty of Medicine
University René Descartes
Paris V, France

and

Rafael F Valle MD
Professor of Obstetrics and Gynecology
Northwestern University Medical School
Chicago, USA

With the assistance of
Fushia Decuypere MD
Port-Royal Hospital, Paris, France

Preface by Rafael F Valle
Drawings by Hubert Guedj

MARTIN DUNITZ

First published in the United Kingdom in 2003
by Martin Dunitz, an imprint of Taylor and Francis,
11 New Fetter Lane, London EC4P 4EE

Tel.:   +44 (0) 20 7583 9855
Fax.:   +44 (0) 20 7842 2298
E-mail: info@dunitz.co.uk
Website: http://www.dunitz.co.uk

A CIP record for this book is available from the British Library

ISBN 1-90186-567-3

Distributed in the USA by
Fulfilment Center
Taylor & Francis
10650 Tobben Drive
Independence, KY 41051, USA
Toll Free Tel: +1 800 634 7064
E-mail: taylorandfrancis@thomsonlearning.com

Distributed in Canada by
Taylor & Francis
74 Rolark Drive
Scarborough, Ontario M1R 4G2, Canada
Toll Free Tel: +1 877 226 2237
E-mail: tal_fran@istar.ca

Distributed in the rest of the world by
Thomson Publishing Services
Cheriton House
North Way
Andover, Hampshire SP10 5BE, UK
Tel: +44 (0)1264 332424
E-mail: salesorder.tandf@thomsonpublishingservices.co.uk

Composition by Scribe Design, Gillingham, Kent
Printed and bound in Singapore by Kyodo Printing Co (S'pore) Pte Ltd

Contents

Preface

A logical step for a physician practicing endoscopy is to use endoscopic methods to treat the abnormal conditions diagnosed. This approach often follows a diagnostic examination. We have compiled this atlas to encompass the various therapeutic procedures that can be performed through hysteroscopy. With this in mind, we have outlined in a concise manner these therapeutic procedures and have illustrated them with superb color pictures that depict important steps in their performance.

In compiling this atlas, we have followed a sequential order to convey to the reader in a didactic manner the different therapeutic modalities performed through the hysteroscope. These operative procedures include those performed with mechanical instruments, those involving the resectoscope with its variously shaped electrodes, and those procedures performed utilizing fiber lasers. Each illustration is accompanied with a legend that helps with the interpretation and places the reader in a specific step and sequence of the operation. Additionally, graphics and sketches for the illustrations have been added to facilitate interpretation.

While therapeutic hysteroscopy is strictly a dynamic process, nonetheless, reviewing pictures provides the gynecologic surgeon with an excellent opportunity to 'caption' a particular step in the chosen procedure, review it at leisure, and understand better the process of performing such a procedure. Furthermore, an atlas comprising color prints permits detailed observation of the various aspects of intrauterine pathology and its resolution by therapeutic hysteroscopy.

These pictures have been generated over many years of experience practicing therapeutic hysteroscopy, and permit the practitioner to review in this volume the various therapeutic procedures that might not be easy to collect in such a manner in a short period of time, even in a busy practice, by a single practitioner. We have attempted to follow a uniform didactic form, maintaining consistency and uniformity.

A concise, yet complete, text is added as an introduction to this atlas, detailing the instrumentation, uterine distending media, indications, and possible complications of operative hysteroscopy. While the text is short and succinct, it includes the basic principles and clinical applications of operative hysteroscopy.

We hope this atlas of *Operative Hysteroscopy* will guide and assist the gynecologist in performing operative hysteroscopy.

Rafael F Valle

Introduction

In only a few years operative hysteroscopy has become very popular among gynecologists, whereas more than a century passed before diagnostic hysteroscopy attained wide acceptance.

At present, with the development of miniaturized cameras, this endoscopic operative technique can be used in the management of all non-cancerous intrauterine lesions, with the entire procedure being performed under video monitoring.

Operative hysteroscopy lends itself very well to the management of leiomyomas, polyps, focal hyperplasia, intrauterine adhesions, uterine malformations, osseous metaplasia, removal of intrauterine devices, and other abnormal intrauterine conditions.

1 Instrumentation

Introduction

Operative hysteroscopy can be performed using three different techniques:

- hysteroscopic scissors inserted into an operative sheath;
- the electrosurgical resectoscope, fitted with various standard electrodes (e.g. a cutting loop for performing resections or the roller-ball or roller-bar of various sizes for coagulation and endometrial ablation); these electrodes are powered by an electric generator with adjustable power settings: 50–100 W modulated current for coagulation and 100–200 W unmodulated current for resection; and
- the neodymium:yttrium aluminum garnet (Nd:YAG) laser, emitting at wavelengths of 1.32 µm.

Hysteroscopic scissors can be used with either liquid or gas distension, but the electrosurgical resectoscope and the Nd:YAG laser can be used only in the presence of a liquid distending medium (1.5% glycine solution for electrosurgery and saline solutions for the laser).

Instruments

Operative hysteroscopes

Operative hysteroscopes (manufactured by Storz, Wolf, Olympus and Circon) have sheaths to accommodate mechanical instruments – scissors, grasping forceps, biopsy forceps, or laser fibers (*Figs 1.1–1.14*).

Multipurpose hysteroscopes accommodate electrodes, mechanical instruments or a laser fiber (e.g. the Baggish hysteroscope manufactured by Bryan) (*Figs 1.15–1.17*). This type of instrument makes use of scissors (*Fig. 1.18*) and three different electrodes: the roller-ball for coagulation (*Fig. 1.19*), a needle-tip for simple cutting (*Fig. 1.20*) and an arch-shaped loop for the resection of small myomas and polyps (*Figs 1.21 and 1.22*). Polyps nestled in a uterine horn

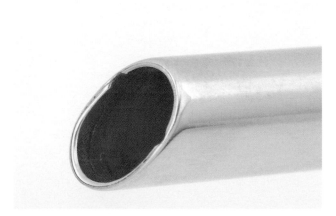

Figure 1.1 Wolf oval cross-section external sheath for operative hysteroscopy.

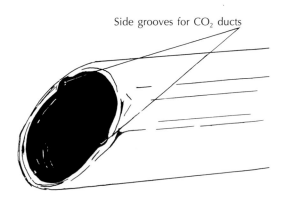

Side grooves for CO_2 ducts

Figure 1.2 Drawing of Fig. 1.1: oval external sheath 8 × 5 mm diameter.

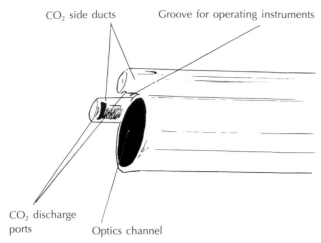

Figure 1.3 Internal sheath with two CO_2 side channels.

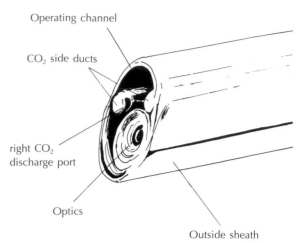

Figure 1.4 Drawing of Fig. 1.7. Assembled operative hysteroscope: lateral view.

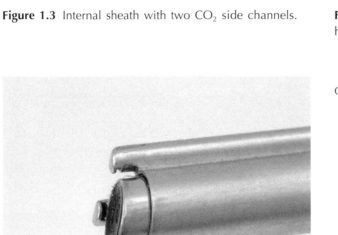

Figure 1.5 Internal sheath with telescope in place; notice the positioning of the gas channel orifice at the end of the telescope.

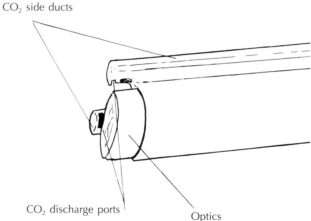

Figure 1.6 Drawing of Fig. 1.5: 4 mm diameter, angle of view 25°.

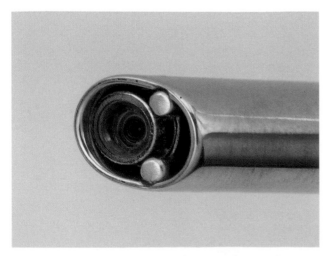

Figure 1.7 Assembled operative hysteroscope ready to accommodate an operating instrument.

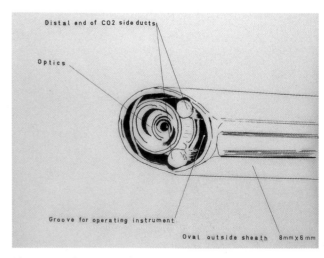

Figure 1.8 Drawing of Fig. 1.7: oval external sheath 8 × 6 mm diameter.

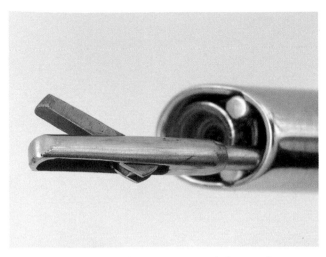

Figure 1.9 Operative hysteroscope with biopsy forceps in place.

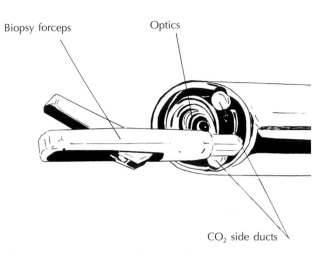

Figure 1.10 Drawing of Fig. 1.9: distal end of operating channel.

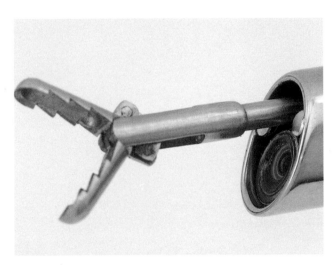

Figure 1.11 Operative hysteroscope with grasping forceps in place.

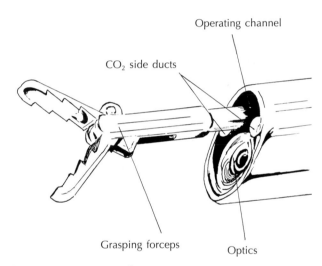

Figure 1.12 Drawing of Fig. 1.11.

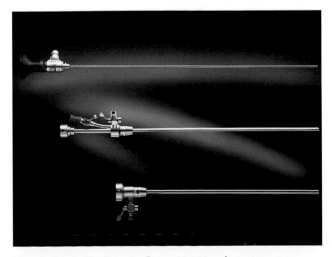

Figure 1.13 Continuous-flow operative hysteroscope; 16 F sheath and 2.7 mm 25° telescope.

Continuous flow operative hysteroscope, 16 Charr.

Telescope PANAVIEW PLUS, 2.7 mm outer diameter
25°...
Inner sheath...
External sheath, round,
16 Charr., useful length, continuous flow,
operative channel 5 Charr..............................

[External small diameter
[Accessories instruments of 5 Char. Maximum
[New appreciably advanced telescope 2.7 mm

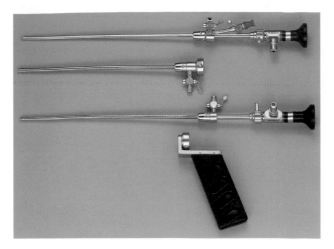

Figure 1.14 Continuous-irrigation ambulatory operative hysteroscope; 15 F compact system with built-in 20° foreoblique lens.

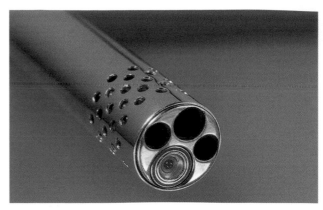

Figure 1.15 Baggish operative hysteroscope: overall view with straightforward lens.

Interchangeable telescope
4 or 2.7 mm

Inner sheath
Operative channel 5 Charr...............................
External sheath, round
16 Char...
Telescope PANAVIEW PLUS
2.7 mm...
Ergonomic handle...

Continuous flow operative hysteroscope 16.5 Charr.

Continuous flow diagnostic hysteroscope 16.5 Charr.

Inner sheath..
External sheath, round..
Telescope PANAVIEW PLUS
4 mm..
Ergonomic handle..

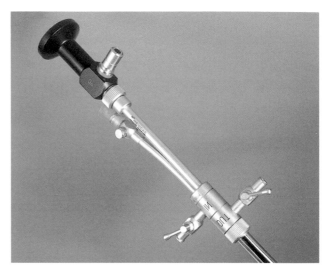

Figure 1.16 Inner sheath with telescope and inflow and outflow stopcocks.

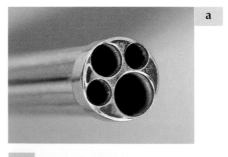

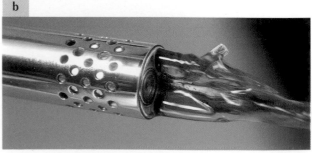

Figure 1.17 (A) End of operative hysteroscope: channel for scissors and double channels for inflow and outflow of liquid. (B) Distending medium.

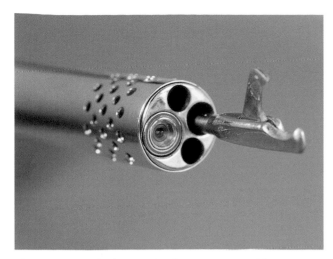

Figure 1.18 End of operative hysteroscope with operative instrument in place: hysteroscopic scissors in the open position.

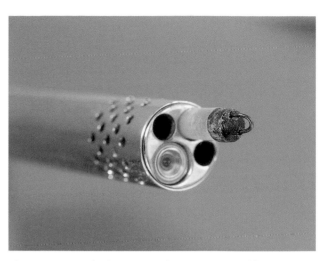

Figure 1.21 End of operative hysteroscope with operative instrument in place: loop electrode in retracted position.

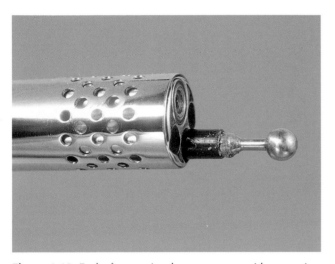

Figure 1.19 End of operative hysteroscope with operative instrument in place: coagulation roller-ball (hemostasis or endometrial ablation).

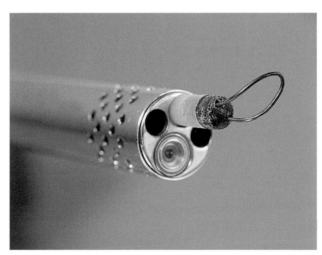

Figure 1.22 End of operative hysteroscope with operative instrument in place: loop electrode in deployed position.

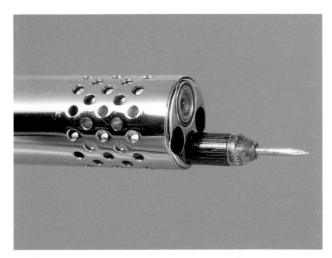

Figure 1.20 End of operative hysteroscope with operative instrument in place: needle-tip electrode for lysing adhesions or sectioning septa.

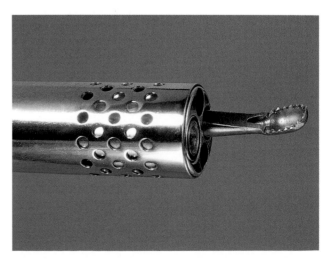

Figure 1.23 End of operative hysteroscope with operative instrument in place: mini-curette for biopsy purposes or for ablation of small polyps.

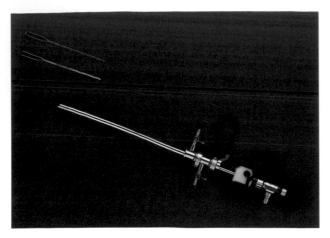

Figure 1.24 Resectoscope.

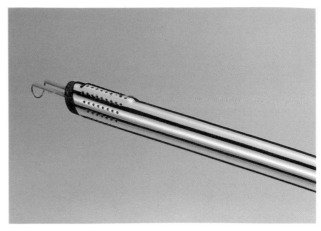

Figure 1.26 Posterior U-shaped loop resection electrode.

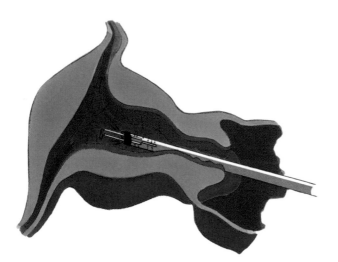

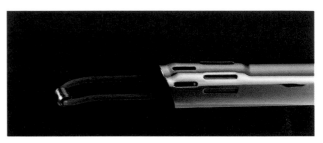

Figure 1.27 Coagulation roller-ball electrode.

Figure 1.25 Dual current resectoscope and unit for continuous irrigation of the uterine cavity; illustration of liquid flow.

are an excellent indication for using this type of instrument (*Figs 1.22 and 1.23*).

The electrosurgical resectoscope

The electrosurgical resectoscope or hysteroresector (manufactured by Storz, Wolf, Olympus and Circon) with continuous irrigation is the instrument best suited for the endoscopic treatment of fibromas and polyps (*Figs 1.24 and 1.25*). It includes:

- a sheath of 27 French–Charr (9 mm), which has fenestrations at its proximal end for controlling the evacuation of the irrigation liquid, ensuring that the uterine cavity is rinsed;
- an inner sheath, whose proximal end controls the infusion of the irrigation liquid;

- an electrode conveyor, which has a mobile handle (site of the thumb) articulated on a V-spring, allowing a back-and-forth movement of the electrode; a fixed, broader handle is used as support at the index and the middle finger (passive mode);
- an arch-shaped cutting loop electrode (*Fig. 1.26*) or a coagulating loop (roller-ball) electrode with a large-surface roller (*Fig. 1.27*);
- a connecting electrical high-frequency cable, 2–4 m in length; and
- an optic of 4 mm diameter with a viewing angle of 25°.

Nd:YAG laser

The Nd:YAG laser is the most effective laser for operative hysteroscopy (*Fig. 1.28*). The laser beams can be transmitted by optical fibers in a liquid distension medium. The amplifying crystal of the Nd:YAG laser includes 20 different transitions providing an emission wavelengh from 0.939 to 1.44 µm. In operative hysteroscopy only a beam of 1.06 µm or 1.32 µm is used (*Fig. 1.29*). The 1.32 µm beam provides a superior cutting effect as well as better hemostasis.

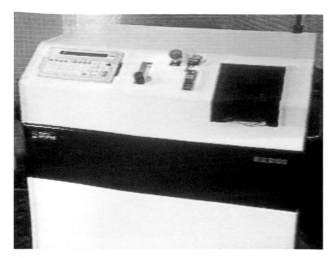

Figure 1.28 Nd:YAG laser.

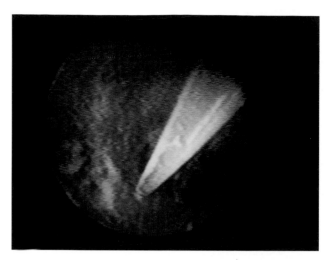

Figure 1.30 Close-up view of the end of a 200 μm diameter laser fiber.

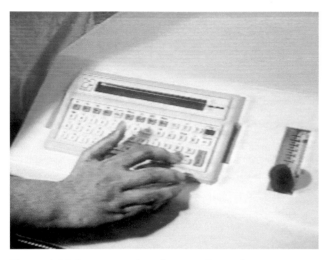

Figure 1.29 Laser wavelength control panel.

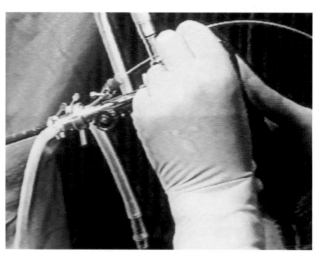

Figure 1.31 Insertion of laser fiber into the operative channel of the hysteroscope.

The tissue effects of the Nd:YAG laser depend on the wavelength used. The wavelengh of 1.06 μm is 100% transmitted by water, and it therefore provides the possibility of remote action. Its main effect is on coagulation and its cutting action is poor. The beam is absorbed preferably by red vascularized tissues.

The wavelength of 1.32 μm is absorbed by water, and it therefore requires the fiber to have contact with the endometrium. The ray has tissue effects which brings it closer to the laser CO_2 where it is more efficiently absorbed: it cuts paler tissues well with limited tissue damage while preserving satisfactory hemostasis. The beam presents less risk than the lower wavelength beam because it is absorbed after crossing tissue if there is water behind. It is absorbed preferably by whitish, hydrated tissues, and its use is indicated in the treatment of fibromas.

The wavelength 1.32 μm is also adapted to the treatment of the uterine septa and the synechiae. Two emission modes are possible:

- pulsatile, which acts on the surface and has a weak diffusion depth of 1.5 mm; and
- continuous, which has greater diffusion depth of 4–5 mm.

The flexible quartz fiber (*Fig. 1.30*) that transmits the beam is introduced into the operative channel of the sheath of the hysteroscope (*Fig. 1.31*); it may be provided with an Albarran bridge, which permits the tip of a flexible instrument to be bent.

Hysteroscopy laser surgery must be performed using protective goggles as backscatter from the beam can damage the surgeon's eye.

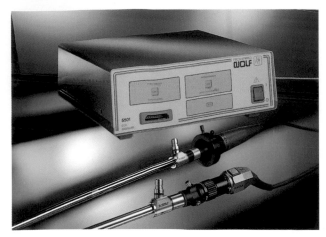

Figure 1.32 Miniaturized video cameras with control unit.

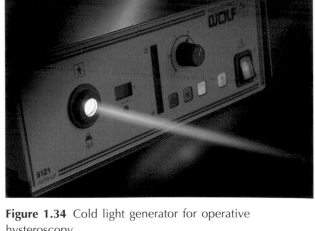

Figure 1.34 Cold light generator for operative hysteroscopy.

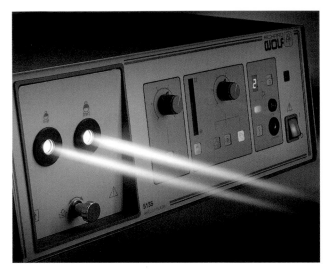

Figure 1.33 Xenon 300 W auto-LP (light projector)–flash light source: light projector for video recording, still photography, and simple observation.

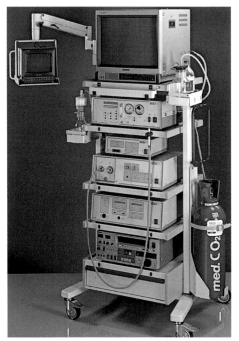

Figure 1.35 General view of operative hysteroscopy equipment and storage cart.

Video instrumentation

Video instrumentation requires:

- a television monitor with a super-fine-pitch trinitron picture tube (with a 0.25 mm aperture grill), which gives high picture resolution – horizontal resolution is more than 600 lines at the center of the picture, and up to 2000 characters can be displayed with great clarity – and Y/C input selection for the signal stream provided by Y/C input leads;
- a miniaturized video camera processor with a sensitivity of light extremely high (3 lux to diaphragm 1.4), with automatic and manual balancing of the white (*Fig. 1.32*); coupled to
- a charge couple device (CCD) video camera head with a waterproof zoom lens, which can be immersed in disinfecting solution and sterilized with gas at temperatures of 60°C; this camera is of small size and light weight (25 g); and
- a cold light generator with a minimum power rating of 400 W (a halogen lamp with arc and metal vapor) and automatic luminosity adjustment according to the video signal (*Figs 1.33 and 1.34*).

The following may optionally be provided:

- a video printer unit to print still color pictures, with memory of up to four images and a thermal-head of resolution 1024 points and 310 dots per inch; and
- a video cassette recorder for intraoperative recording on video tape.

The video equipment can be mounted on a small cart with wheels for easy maneuverability (*Fig. 1.35*).

Distending media

Gaseous media

CO_2 is used under rigorously controlled flow rate and intrauterine pressure; these conditions are monitored by a reliable flowmeter (*Fig. 1.36*). The maximum permissible flow rate is 100 ml/minute and the maximum permissible intrauterine pressure is 150 mmHg.

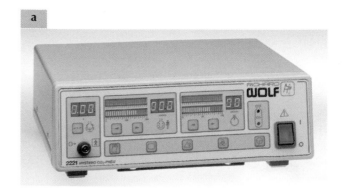

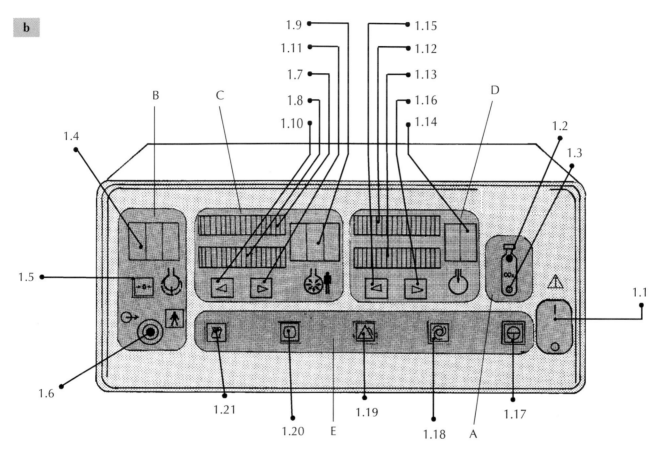

1.1 Power switch

A Gas reserve
1.2 Gas reserve (green light indicator of unit operating)
1.3 Residual gas amber light indicator

B Consumption of gas
1.4 Digital display of quantity of used gas
1.5 Reset button
1.6 Connection of insufflation rubber tubing

C Manometric control
1.7 Warning light of effective intra uterine pressure
1.8 Warning light of preselected pressure
1.9 Intra uterine pressures digital display
1.10 Pressure decrease
1.11 Pressure increase

D Gas flow rate control
1.12 Warning light of effective gas
1.13 Warning light of preselected flow rate gas
1.14 Gas flow rates digital display
1.15 Gas flow rate reduction (down)
1.16 Gas flow rate increase (up)

E Specific functions
1.17 Open-close insufflation function
1.18 Function in automatic mode
1.19 Alarm light indicator
1.20 Video visualization
1.21 Printing button

Figure 1.36 (a,b) Pneumatic CO_2 insufflator: this new-generation instrument is microprocessor-controlled and has digital preselection of desired intrauterine pressure and gas flow rate.

However, because of the risk of gas embolism under general anesthesia (three gas embolisms occurred in 5140 hysteroscopies under general anesthesia performed in 42 centers, giving an incidence of 0.58 per 1000), CO_2 is not used in operative hysteroscopy. It remains the preferable medium of distension for diagnostic hysteroscopy performed without anesthesia and must be replaced by physiological saline solution when the procedure is performed under anesthesia.

Liquid media

The instillation pressure is approximately 100 mmHg. Operative hysteroscopy requires the use of low-viscosity solutions, which offer the best working conditions. These solutions allow continuous irrigation of the uterine cavity through a double-current device that continuously renews the distension liquid and maintains the transparency of the medium.

Distilled water can be used. Its advantages include its low cost, efficient electric section and coagulation, its good transparency, and (in the absence of bleeding) its easy handling. Unfortunately it risks hemolysis in prolonged use. Therefore an aqueous solution with sufficient osmotic pressure to avoid this phenomenon is needed.

Electrolyte-containing solutions

Sodium chloride solution (0.9%)
When infused continuously at a pressure level sufficient to distend the uterine cavity, sodium chloride (NaCl) solution allows very good viewing of the uterine cavity. In the event of vascular intravasation, NaCl will not penetrate into the cells. Because 0.9% sodium chloride solution is isotonic and isomolar, it does not causes hemolysis. Except when electrosurgery is involved, this solution is highly recommended, owing to its absence of toxicity.

Isotonic lactated Ringer solution
Isotonic lactated Ringer solution possesses the same qualities and advantages as 0.9% sodium chloride solution. Because its electrolytic make-up is closer to that of the extracellular fluid, it causes less disruption to the acid–base balance.

Non-electrolyte solutions
No non-electrolyte solution has really proved its superiority, and the choice depends on the practices of each operator.

Dextrose solution (5%)
Dextrose solution is readily available and inexpensive, and it provides clear viewing of the uterine cavity and permits electrosurgery, which is not possible with saline solution. Its drawback is the formation of residue on the optic of the instrument caused by the 'caramelization' effect of electric current on the sugar.

Sorbitol solution (3%)
Sorbitol solution (3%) is a non-electrolytic solution, electrically non-conductive and with an osmolarity of 165 mOsmol/Liter. Because it is a reduced form of dextrose, it is metabolized to carbon dioxide and water and/or excreted by a normally functioning kidney.

Mannitol solution (5%)
Mannitol 5% is an inert substance with 270 mOsmol/Liter osmolarity that acts as a diuretic and helps in the removal of free water, should excessive amounts have been absorbed. About 6–10% of the absorbed Mannitol is metabolized and the remainder is filtered by the kidney. The half-life of Mannitol in the plasma is 15 minutes. However, being an intravascular osmol, when administered, it may increase the intravascular volume as well.

Glycine solution (1.5%)
Glycine is the least complex amino acid in the human body. It is widely used in aqueous solution by urologists for vesicular and prostate gland resection, and it is also used by a growing number of gynecologists. A non-hemolytic, highly diluted 1.5% solution is used to reduce the quantity of glycine absorbed during intravasation.

During the operative procedure, serum electrolytes, especially sodium, must be very carefully monitored because glycine solution may cause metabolic problems as a result of the absence of electrolytes in the solution. For this reason, the flow rate and pressure of the solution should be controlled, either by using an infusion pump or by hanging the bag on an infusion pole.

Flexible chloride, polyvinyl, plasticized bags containing 3 liters of solution are used (*Fig. 1.37*). Using two bags twinned with a Siamese connection makes it possible to infuse 6 liters continuously without needing to change the bag.

The infusion pump is an electrical roller-action hysteroscopic pump, that ensures the distension and continuous irrigation of the uterine cavity (Fig. 1.38). The propulsion of the liquid is ensured by the rotation of a roller that compresses a portion of flexible piping

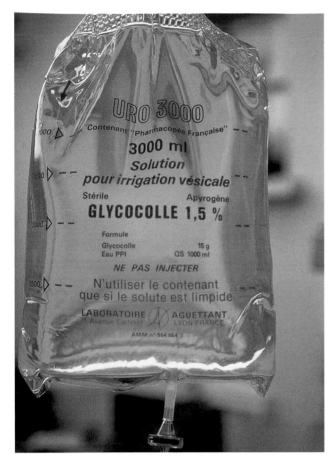

Figure 1.37 Plastic bag of 1.5% glycine solution.

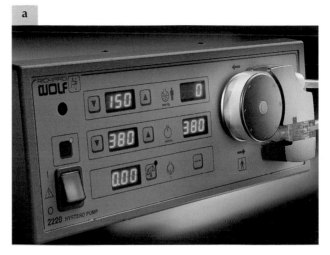

1 Power switch and indicator
2 Pump open-close button
3 Remote control sensor
4 Preselected pressure button: decrease (down)
5 Preselected pressure digital display
6 Preselected pressure button: increase (up)
7 Effective pressure digital display
8 Room of compression switch
9 Pump head with pressure sensors
10 Roller pump
11 Effective flow rate display
12 Preselected flow rate button: increase (up)
13 Preselected flow rate digital display
14 Preselected flow rate button: decrease (down)
15 Reset button
16 Balance button
17 Volume digital display

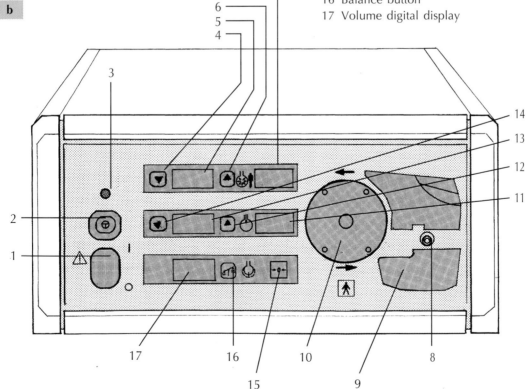

Figure 1.38 (a,b) Glycine hysteropump featuring built-in balancing of quantity of liquid, infrared remote control, and printer interface port allowing immediate recording of all data from the intervention. (b) Drawing of (a).

connecting the bag to the hysteroscope. A compression chamber integrated into the flexible piping and fixed at the pump transmits electronically through sensors, the pressure reigning in piping with a regulating system of pressure.

The desired pressure is preselected with regard to the safe limits and the effective pressure is automatically provided by the pump. When the effective pressure exceeds the selected pressure, the regulating circuit reverses the direction of rotation of the roller and reduces the pressure. If in spite of this regulation, the pressure exceeds the safety threshold planned for the pump, and it stops automatically.

The maximum flow rate also is preselected. Visual and sound alarms are available when the threshold is exceeded.

The pressure usually selected for an operation does not exceed 150 mmHg; the flow rate may range from 300 to 450 ml/minute. The total volume delivered can also be indicated by the pump.

It is important to purge the system of air well before its placement in the uterine cavity, because bubbles of air represent a potential cause of gas embolism.

2 Indications

Abnormal uterine bleeding

Polypectomy

For a long time the extraction of the polyps was done by curettage, and numerous failures resulted from the blind nature of this technique. The advent of operative hysteroscopy represented considerable progress, because the procedure could be carried out under visual control.

Uterine polyps are generally mucous – they are localized excrescences of uterine mucosa consisting of glands and stroma around a vascular axis (*Figs 2.1–2.3*). They often occur in the context of a hormonal disorder (e.g. dysovulation, corpus luteal insufficiency, hyperestrogenism). They are most common in women aged between 40 and 50 years. Their size varies from a few millimeters in diameter

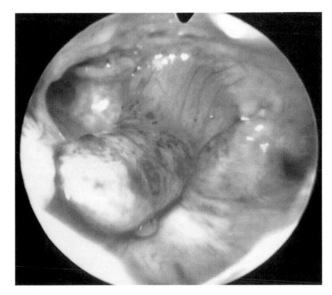

Figure 2.1 A broad-based pedunculated endometrial polyp located on the uterine fundus.

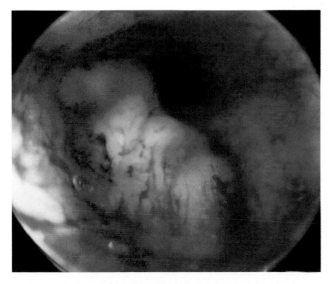

Figure 2.2 A sessile endocervical polyp.

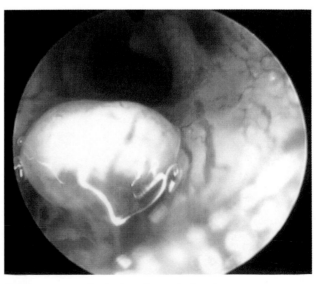

Figure 2.3 A spherical endocervical polyp.

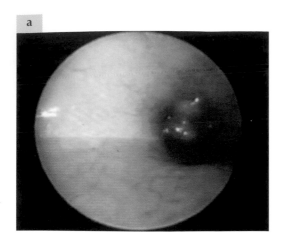

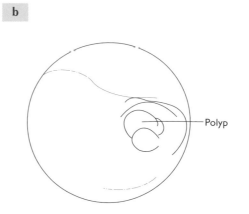

Figure 2.4 (a,b) Small polyp in the left uterine horn: this is a classic indication for using the Baggish retractable loop hysteroscope.

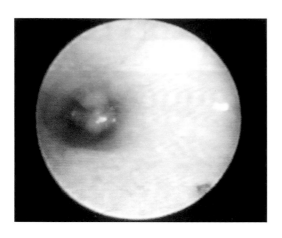

Figure 2.5 Close-up view of right uterine horn, showing two small polyps obstructing the tubal ostium. The electric loop can be used if its electric loop is of small diameter. The electric loop of the Baggish hysteroscope finds one of its best indications here.

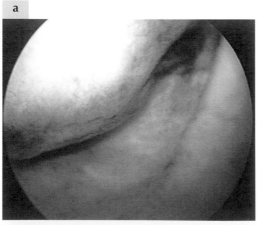

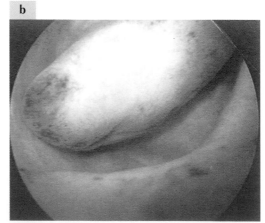

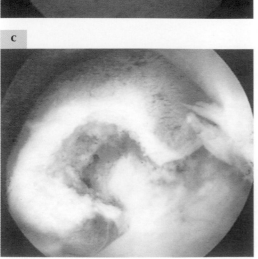

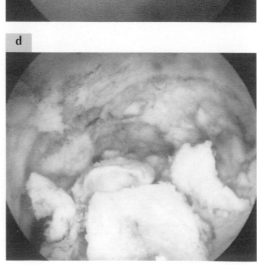

Figure 2.6 Polypectomy with resectoscope: the pedunculated polyp is located on the left uterine horn. (a,b) Before resection; (c) during resection; (d) after resection.

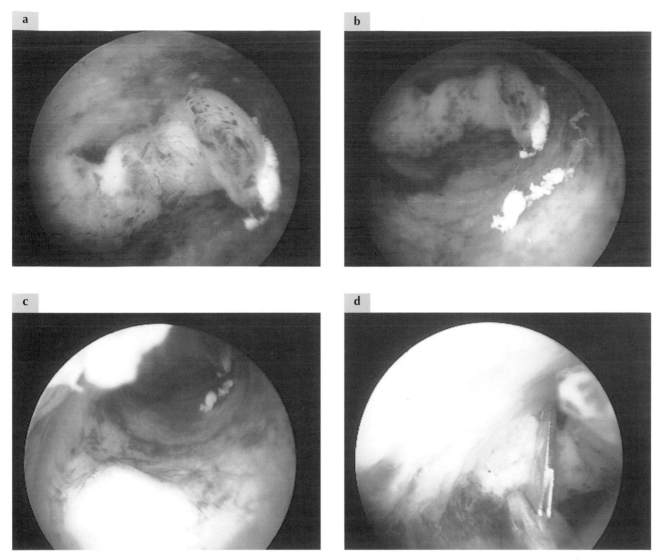

Figure 2.7 (a–d) Sectioning by scissors in liquid medium of a pedunculated polyp located on the right side of the uterus.

(*Figs 2.4 and 2.5*) to bulky masses occupying the whole uterine cavity and measuring 8–10 cm in diameter (*Fig. 2.6*).

Pedunculated polyps are extracted by sectioning the pedicle of the polyp with scissors in a liquid or gaseous medium (*Figs 2.8 and 2.10; see also Fig. 2.5*) or by using a resectoscope (*see Fig. 2.6*).

Sessile polyps are ablated by resection with a 28 F resector in a liquid medium. The polyp is withdrawn *en bloc* or in several fragments with an electric loop or a curette (*Fig. 2.9*).

Hysteroscopy can reveal whether an endometrial polyp is functional or non-functional.

Functional polyps
In about half of the cases, polyps are functional and the patient's only symptom is menorrhagia.

Functional polyps tend to be single and not very large (2–5 mm in diameter), and their color and the distribution of blood vessels on their surface is like that of the adjacent endometrium.

Functional polyps are often sessile, although some are pedunculated with a short, thick pedicle. They look linguiform (*Fig. 2.12*), triangular or coniform. A trickle of blood is visible in some cases from hematomas on the tip of the polyp.

Functional sessile polyps can be curetted, but it is necessary to repeat the hysteroscopic observation to evaluate the effect of therapy, because a functional polyp that has been confirmed histologically by curettage may not be removed completely even after menstruation. For this reason, the removal of these polyps is more effective by resectoscopic resection (*Fig. 2.13 and see Fig. 2.2*).

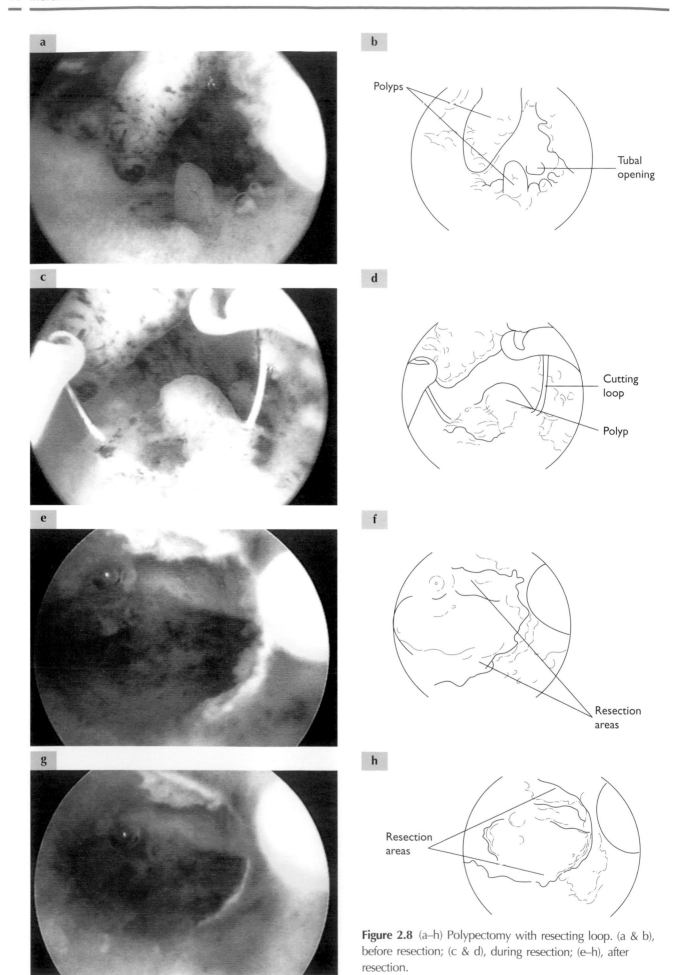

Figure 2.8 (a–h) Polypectomy with resecting loop. (a & b), before resection; (c & d), during resection; (e–h), after resection.

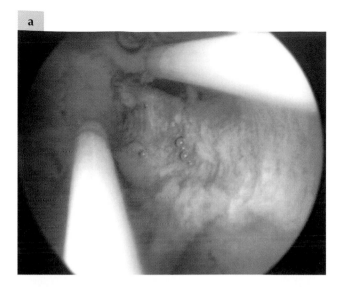

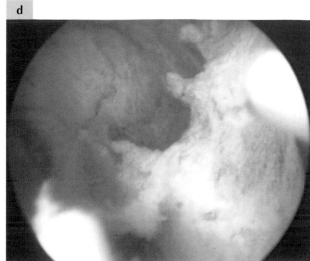

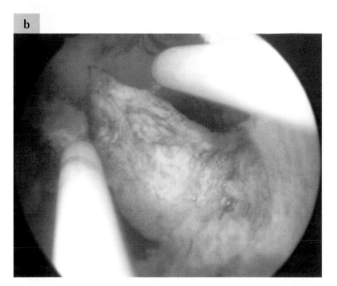

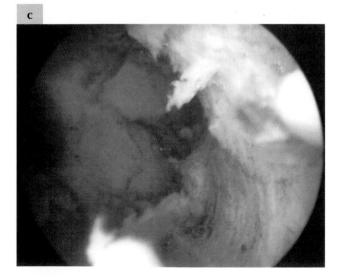

Figure 2.9 Four steps in the resection of a polyp: the resectoscopic cutting loop is placed behind the polyp and drawn back toward the hysteroscopic sheath.

Non-functional polyps

Non-functional polyps are the most common type of polyp. Patients have abnormal uterine bleeding – menorrhagia or metrorrhagia in women of child-bearing age (glandular hyperplastic polyps) or postmenopausal spotting in older women (adenomatous polyps). Non-functional polyps vary in size, but they can be large. They are more regular in shape (round or oval), and harder than functional polyps, and they are yellow–red in color (*Fig. 2.14*). Subepithelial vessels are rarely visible and the overlying mucosa is thick. They may be sessile or pedunculated. These polyps are removed by resectoscopic resection (*Fig. 2.15*).

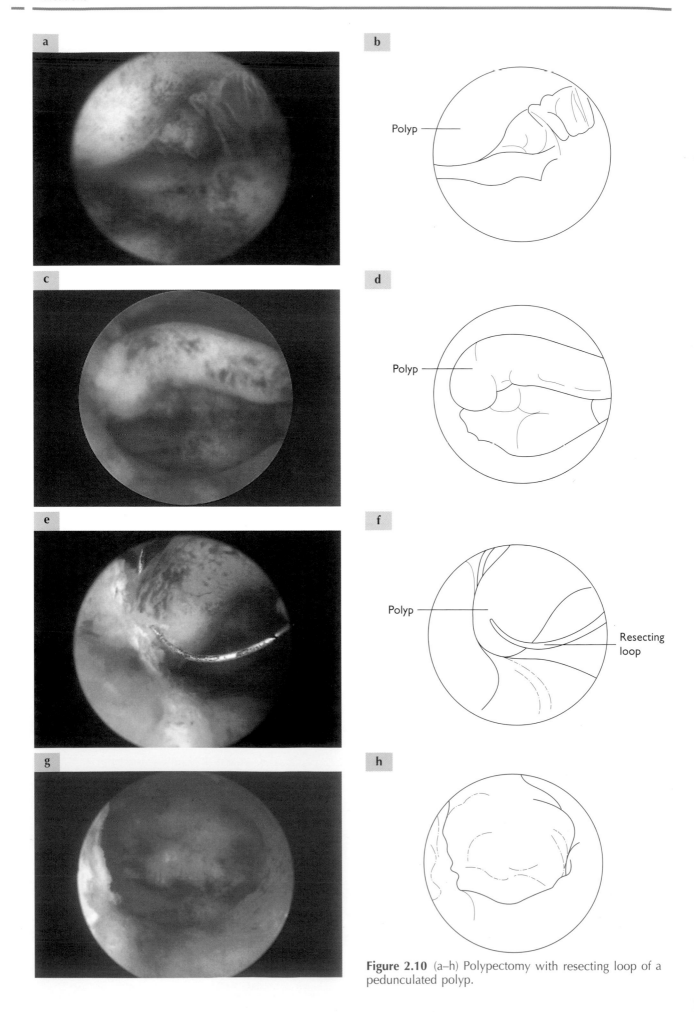

Figure 2.10 (a–h) Polypectomy with resecting loop of a pedunculated polyp.

a

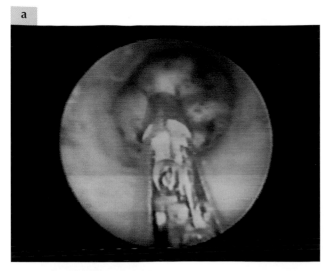

Figure 2.11 Removal of polyp with forceps.

b

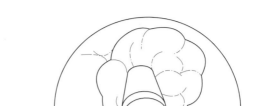

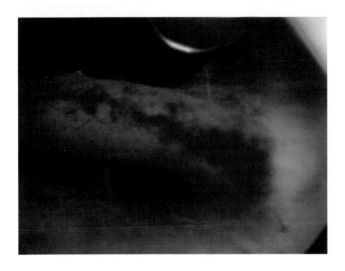

Figure 2.12 Linguiform aspect of the functional polyp, with hematomas on the edge. The color and blood vessel distribution on the surface of the polyp are similar to those of the adjacent endometrium.

Myomectomy

Sessile or pedunculated leiomyomas are the most frequently encountered indication for operative hysteroscopy (*Figs 2.16 and 2.17*). Twenty per cent of intra uterine lesions are myomas. Submucosal growth of the myoma such that it protrudes into the uterine cavity and causes substantial bleeding is an indication for myomectomy (*Fig. 2.18*).

Submucous myomas are treated on an outpatient basis by operative hysteroscopy, followed by a short period of convalescence. Interstitial and subserosal myomas do not warrant medical or surgical treatment of any kind unless their volume is such that it prevents pregnancy or causes abnormal uterine bleeding. The more serious submucous myoma derives benefit from the new types of endoscopic treatments.

The first step in endoscopic treatment of a myoma is hemostasis of the large blood vessels on the surface (*Figs 2.19–2.24*) or pedicle of the tumor under visual control. The protruding portion of the myoma is removed by shaving it into slices by directing the wire loop beyond the myoma and cutting towards the operator. The cutting movement must always be performed from the fundus towards the isthmus (*Figs 2.25–2.31*). Coagulation is performed, after rinsing the cavity, by opening the stopcock to the glycine solution.

Pedunculated fibromas can be treated by scissors sectioning (*Figs 2.32–2.35*) or by Nd:YAG laser ablation (*Fig. 2.36*). Removal of the cuttings is the most tedious part of the procedure. The large cumbersome cuttings can be removed by grasping them between the wire loop and the tip of the optics and then withdrawing them one by one.

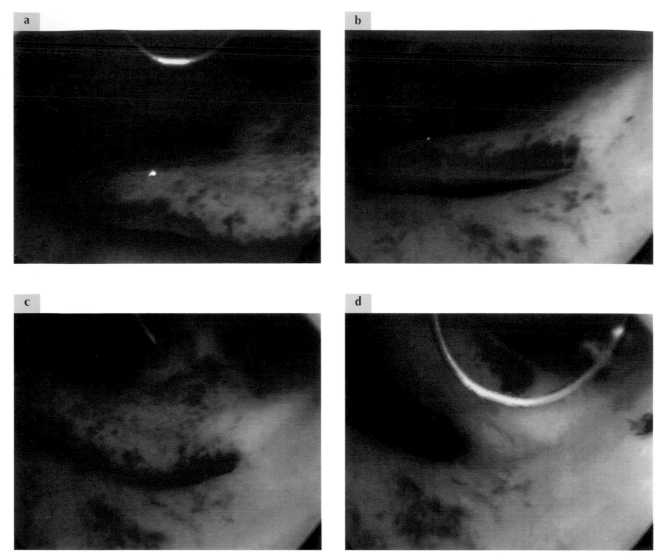

Figure 2.13 (a–d) Resectoscopic resection is the procedure of choice for removal of a functional polyp.

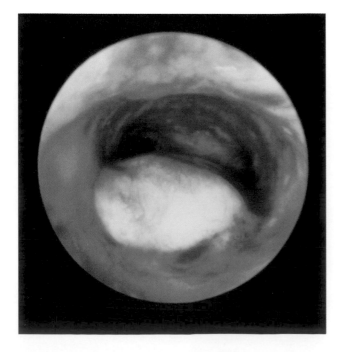

Figure 2.14 Non-functional polyp with a broad implantation on posterior wall, yellow–red in color.

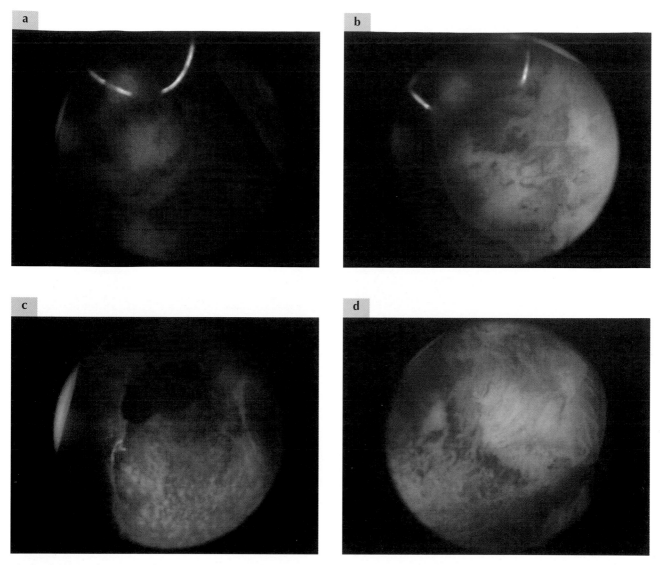

Figure 2.15 (a–d) Stages of resection of a non-functional polyp (adenomatous polyp).

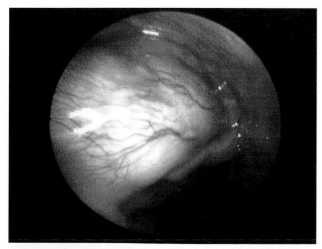

Figure 2.16 Pedunculated fibroma located on the left uterine cornu.

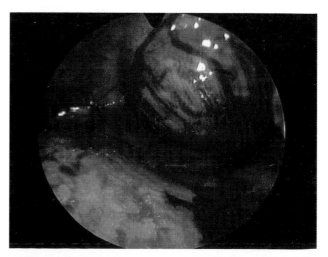

Figure 2.17 Sessile fibroma arising from the anterior wall of the uterus; it represents only a portion of the entire myoma, which is largely intramural.

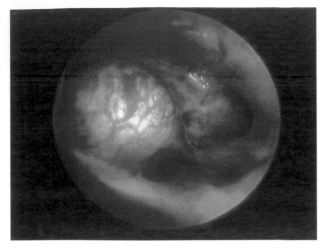

Figure 2.18 Appearance before coagulation. Submucosal myoma with an extensive vascular pattern.

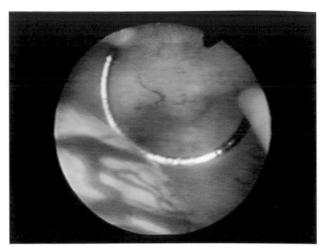

Figure 2.19 Start of coagulation: positioning of the loop electrode; numerous vessels are clearly visible.

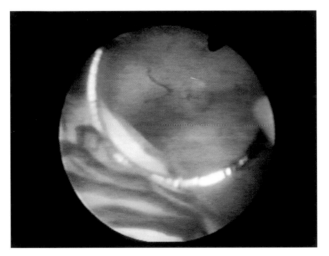

Figure 2.20 During coagulation: the resectoscope allows the electric loop to contact the surface of the fibroma creating a whitening of the vessels.

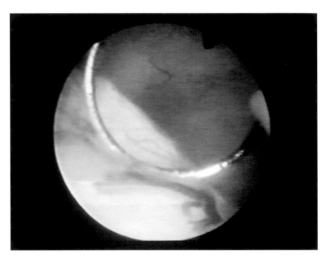

Figure 2.21 End of coagulation: the surface vessels are almost entirely whitish.

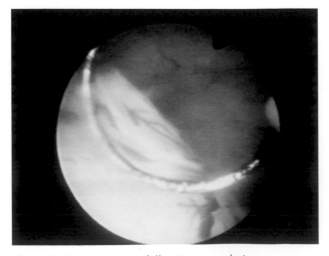

Figure 2.22 Appearance following coagulation.

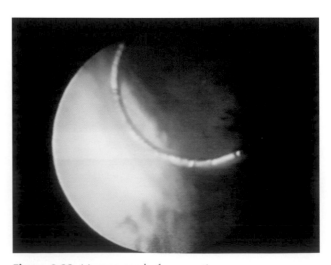

Figure 2.23 Myoma ready for resection.

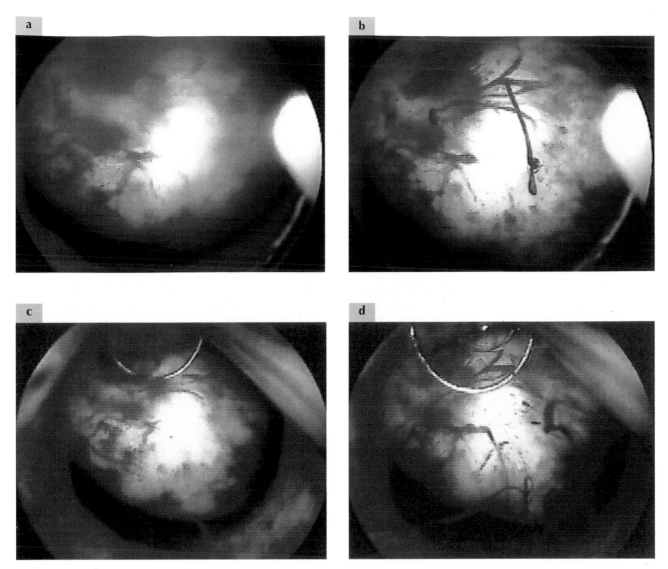

Figure 2.24 Operative hysteroscopy: resection of a submucous myoma. The resecting loop coagulates the surface vessels before resection of the myoma.

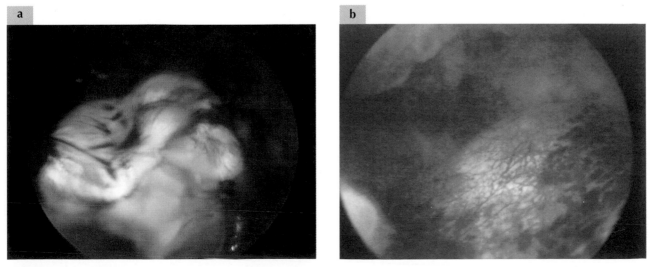

Figure 2.25 (contd).

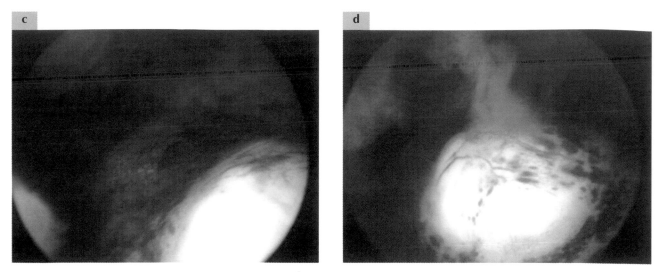

Figure 2.25 (a–d) Large sessile submucous myoma on the posterior wall before resection. (a) submucous myoma shows surface vascular pattern, causing bleeding; (c–d) the sessile myoma occupies the complete posterior wall and extends to both cornu.

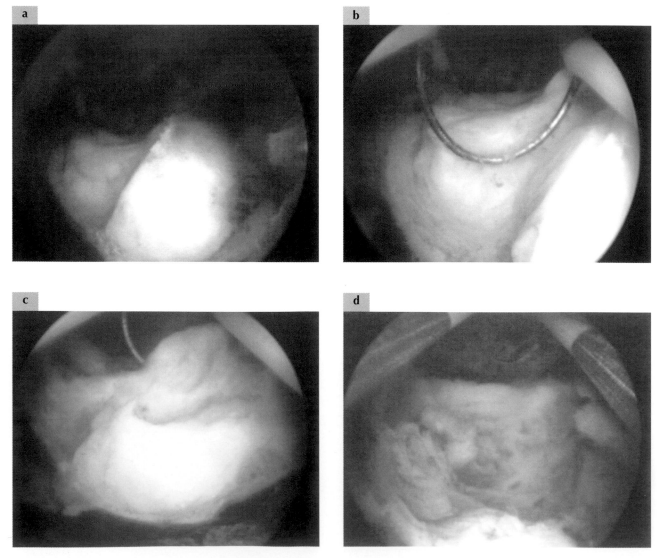

Figure 2.26 Operative hysteroscopy in the same patient as in Fig. 2.25: four steps in the resection of a submucous myoma located on the posterior uterine wall.

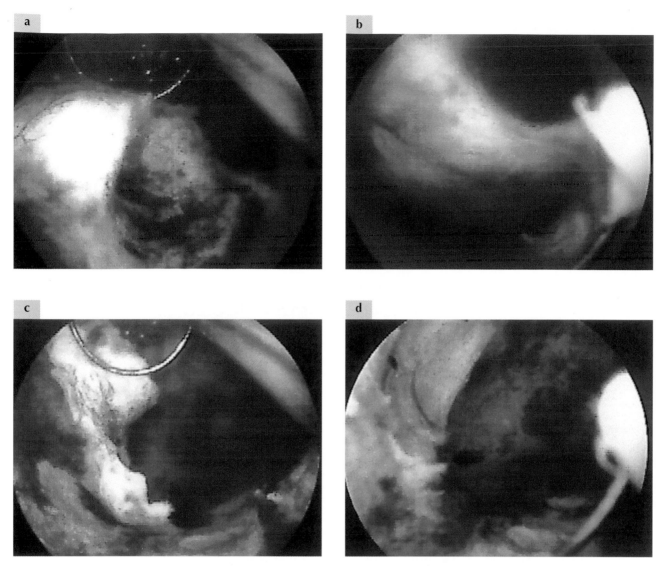

Figure 2.27 Operative hysteroscopy: resection of a submucous myoma. (a) The resecting cutting loop is placed at the back of the myoma and is engaged. (b) First furrow hollowed on the left side of the myoma; then the procedure is repeated up until the base of the pedicle. (c) End of resection: the base of the pedicle is resected level with surrounding endometrium. (d) Aspect of right uterine cornu: the ostium is now accessible.

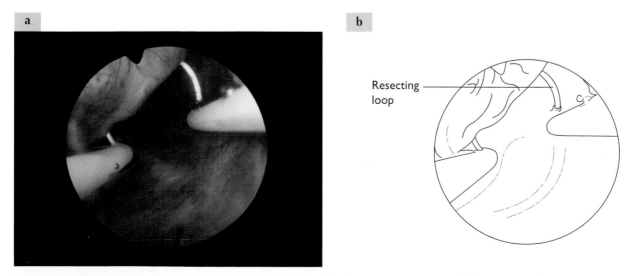

Figure 2.28 Resection of a sessile myoma on posterior wall of uterus: positioning of the resection loop.

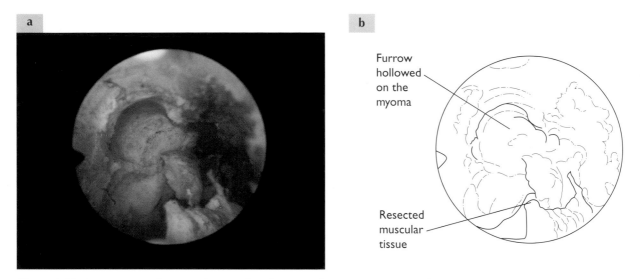

Figure 2.29 During resection: detachment of part of the sessile myoma.

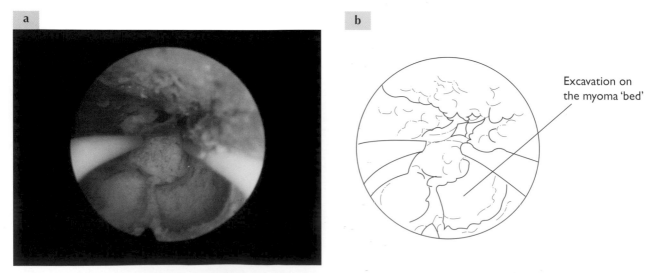

Figure 2.30 Appearance of resected area after the procedure to resect a sessile myoma.

Figure 2.31 Resection can be continued beneath the myoma 'bed': excavation into the intramural portion of a sessile myoma.

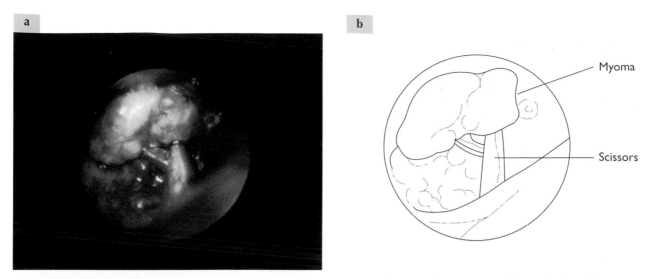

Figure 2.32 Scissors ablation of a myoma on the posterior uterine wall: start of sectioning of the pedicle of the myoma.

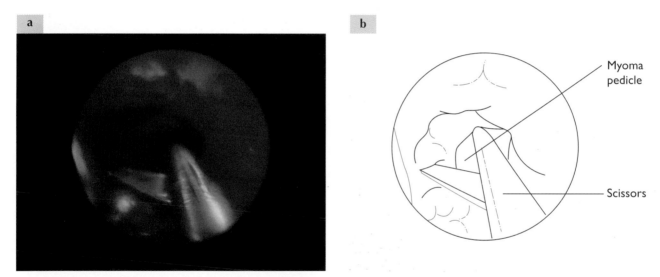

Figure 2.33 Scissors ablation of myoma on the posterior uterine wall: end of procedure (removal of pedicle attachment area).

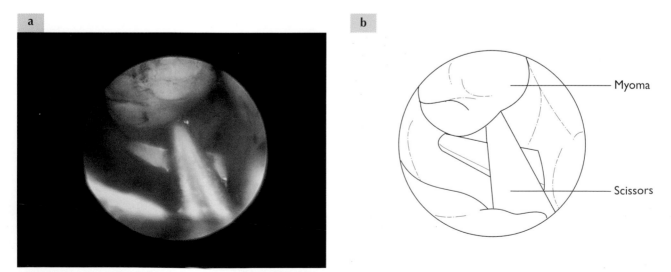

Figure 2.34 Scissors ablation of a myoma on the anterior uterine wall: start of sectioning of the pedicle of the myoma.

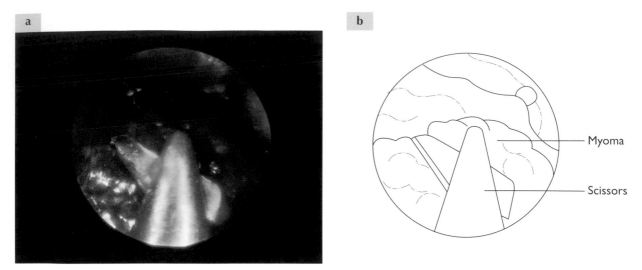

Figure 2.35 Scissors ablation of a myoma on the anterior uterine wall: end of procedure (removal of pedicle attachment area).

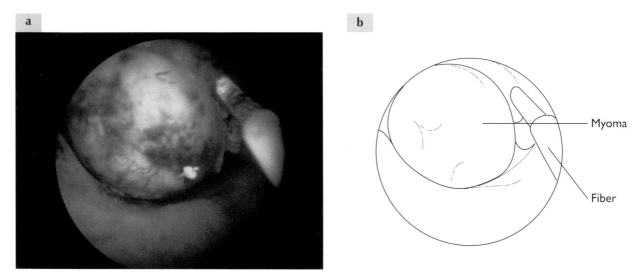

Figure 2.36 Myomectomy of a pedunculated myoma with an Nd:YAG laser (wavelength 1.32 μm).

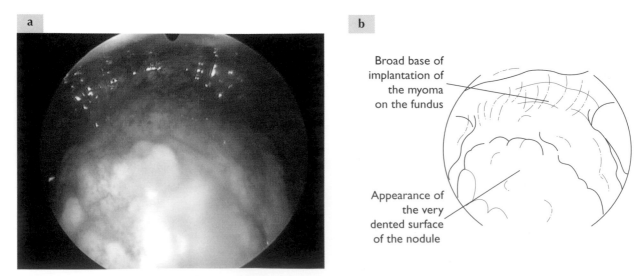

Figure 2.37 Anterior view of myoma, revealing its broad base of implantation.

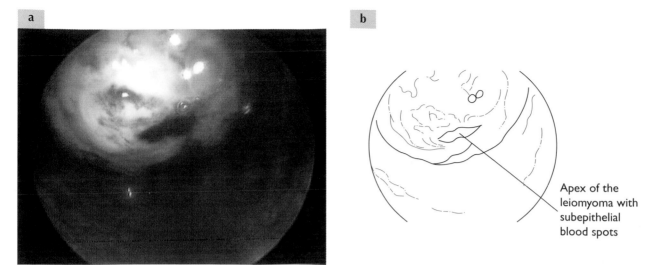

Figure 2.38 Posterior view of the myoma in Fig. 2.37.

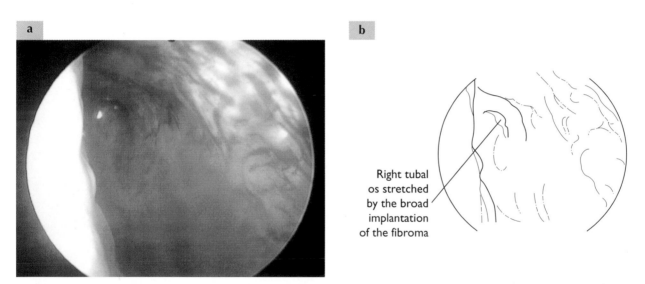

Figure 2.39 View of the right side of the myoma in Fig. 2.37, showing its proximity to the right tubal os.

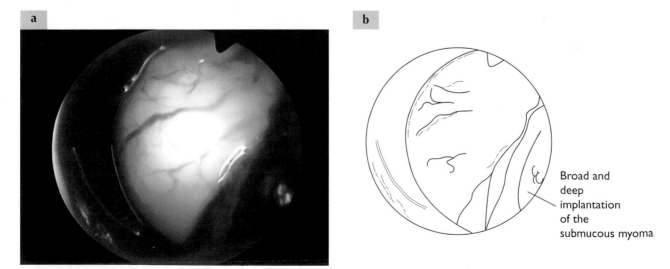

Figure 2.40 A large submucous myoma on the posterior wall and left edge of the uterus. Intraoperative ultrasound revealed the extent of intramural penetration.

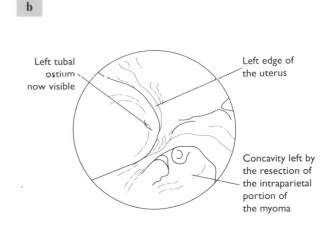

Figure 2.41 Result 3 months following resection of the myoma in Fig. 2.40, showing the excavation left by the intraparietal portion of the resected myoma.

When a part of the myoma is intramural and so embedded to a greater or lesser degree into the uterine wall, the intramural part, which tends to disintegrate either during the procedure or postoperatively, must be ablated if it is left *in situ* (*see Figs 2.28–2.31*). To avoid perforation, care must be taken not to resect too deeply. Therefore preoperative ultrasound is extremely useful and informative in the case of hemispherical myomas that are half interstitial and half submucosal. When the ultrasound examination is performed properly by a vaginal and suprapubic approach, it will reveal the size and location of the lesion as well as the growth of its interstitial portion compared with the intrauterine portion. Injury to juxtaposed structures can occur if the instrument penetrates the myometrium, so care must be taken by 'a wall of security myometrium' to avoid perforation. The echographic examination can disclose the thickness of the 'security' myometrium. This information is extremely useful in guiding the intramural resection procedure so as to avoid perforation (*Figs 2.37–2.41*).

The Nd:YAG laser can also be used (*see Fig. 2.36*) on the intramural portion of the myoma by inducing necrosis. A wavelength of 1.06 μm and 40 W power is used. Destruction induced by the laser can reach 3–4 mm beyond the point of impact. Abdominal or better rectal ultrasound can be used as parapet. The shootings will have set out again all the 2 or 3 millimeters. The informations provided then by preoperative ultrasound are very significant thus. A good evaluation of thickness of the myometrium between the deep surface of the fibroma and the external surface of the uterus avoids going too far or too dangerously.

In short, then, pedunculated myomas can be withdrawn in a semicomplete way. Submucous and interstitial hemispherical myomas can leave a more or less significant residual portion. Hemorrhage may cease but a control hysteroscopy will be necessary 3 months later, and reintervention may be needed.

Small fibromas that are difficult to access because they are in a uterine horn can benefit from the use of photocoagulation with Nd:YAG laser, which brings about necrosis, leaving the fibroma in place but also preserving the tubal ostium in a woman who wishes to become pregnant. The resector can be used if its electric loop is of small diameter (15 F). The electric loop of the Baggish hysteroscope is especially useful here (*Fig. 2.42*). However, if the submucous myoma bulging in the uterine horn is too big, its resection is more difficult and dangerous because of the thinness of the cornual area and the high risk of perforation (*Fig. 2.43*).

Fibromas of moderate size that are well encapsulated can be extirpated with the electric loop of the resectoscope, which is used like a lever or a push rod without using the electric power (*Figs 2.44 and 2.45*). The fibroma is then extracted entirely from its bed and is withdrawn using a grasping forceps.

Contraindications to hysteroscopic myomectomy are:

- exceedingly large submucosal myomas (*Fig. 2.46*);
- myoma embedded in one of the uterine horns (*Figs 2.43 and 2.47*); and
- uterine polymyomatosis (*Fig. 2.48*).

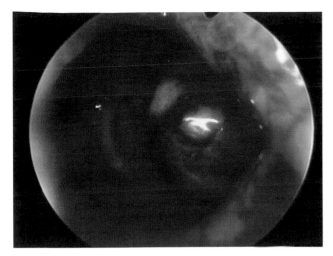

Figure 2.42 Small sessile fibroma huddled in the left uterine horn: the resector can be used if its electric loop is of small diameter.

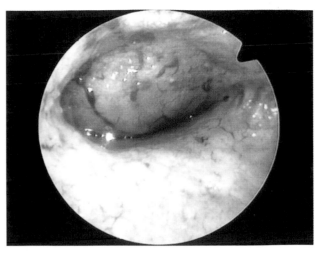

Figure 2.43 This submucous myoma is bulging into the right uterine horn: its resection is more difficult and dangerous because of the thinness of the cornual area and the high risk of perforation (same patient as in Fig. 2.47).

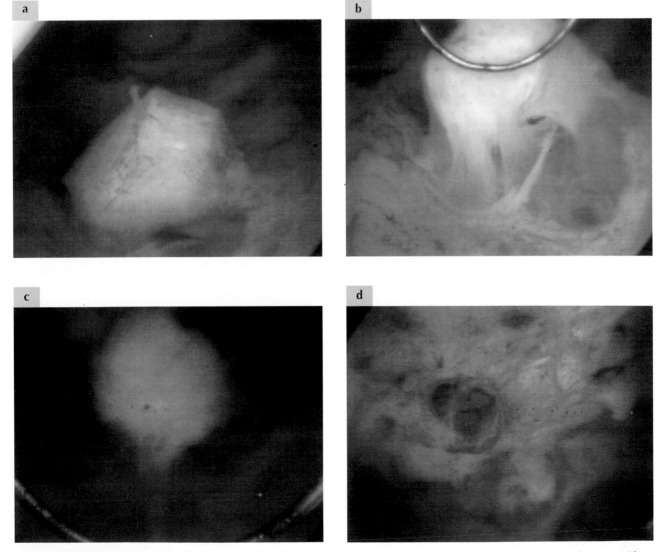

Figure 2.44 (a,b) Enucleation of a small sessile submucous myoma on the posterior wall with the cutting loop. (c) The myoma is almost removed. (d) After enucleation, the fibroma is completely removed from its bed.

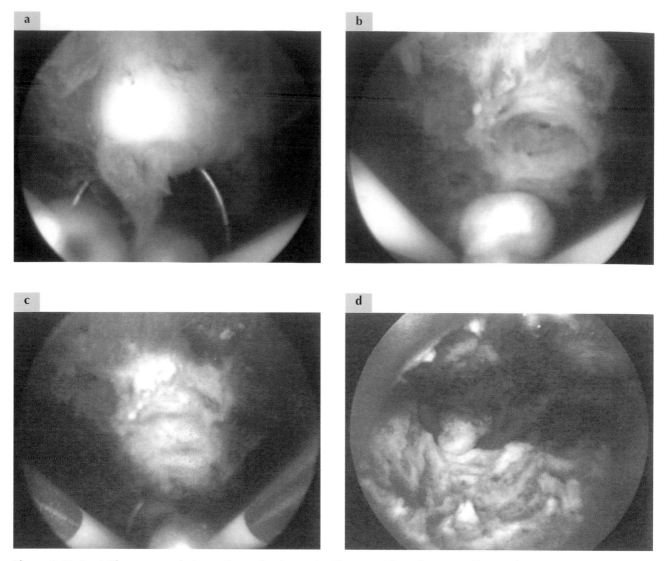

Figure 2.45 (a–c) The same technique of enucleation as in Fig. 2.44 of a submucous fibroma located on the anterior wall of the uterus. (d) Endometrial ablation of the posterior wall.

Endometrial ablation

Endometrial ablation is performed by resection using an electric wire loop, by coagulation using the 'roller-ball' or by photocoagulation with the Nd:YAG laser (1.06 μm in a liquid medium). This procedure corrects recurrent metrorrhagia that is unresponsive to hormonal treatment in premenopausal and perimenopausal women who have no organic uterine lesions. It is an alternative to hysterectomy.

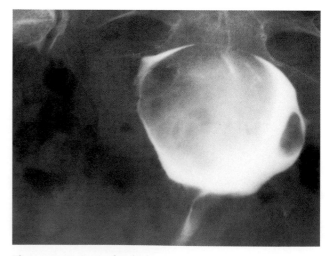

Figure 2.46 Exceedingly large submucosal myoma.

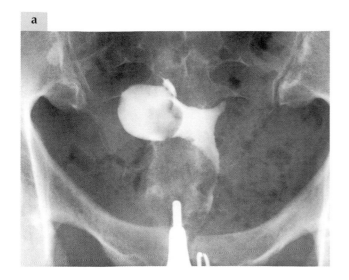

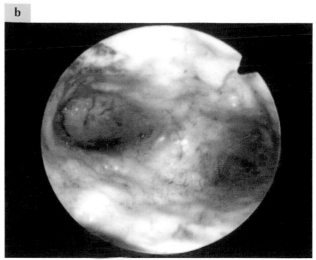

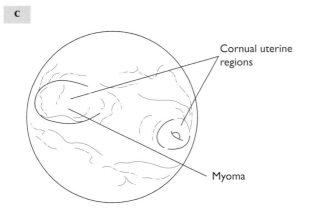

Cornual uterine regions

Myoma

Figure 2.47 Myoma embedded in one of the uterine horns. (a) hysterographic view; (b) hysteroscopic view; (c) drawing.

Indications

Endometrial ablation is indicated in:

- hemorrhagic menstrual disorders (menorrhagia, metrorrhagia); and
- uterine bleeding caused by dysfunctional or benign organic endometrial disorders (endometrial hyperplasia, subatrophic endometrium, superficial adenomyosis).

It should not be proposed in young women, even those who do not wish to remain fertile. It should be reserved for women aged over 40 years. After the menopause, endometrial ablation is indicated in metrorrhagia in patients on hormone replacement therapy after neoplasia has been ruled out by directed biopsies of the endometrium.

Endometrial ablation is contraindicated in patients with a large uterus (of more than 10 cm in diameter), in patients with a polyfibromatous uterus, and in patients with deep diverticular adenomyosis that is visible hysterographically.

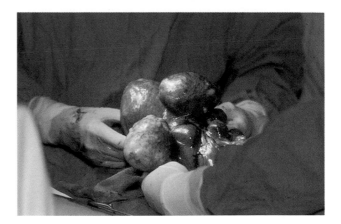

Figure 2.48 Uterine polymyomatosis: operative field.

Technique

For the operation to be successful, the endometrium must be entirely destroyed, along with the basal layer and the first few millimeters of the myometrium. Endometrial ablation thus destroys the

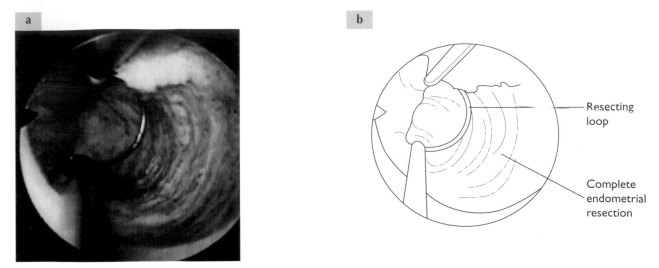

Figure 2.49 Loop resection of the left side of the posterior uterine wall.

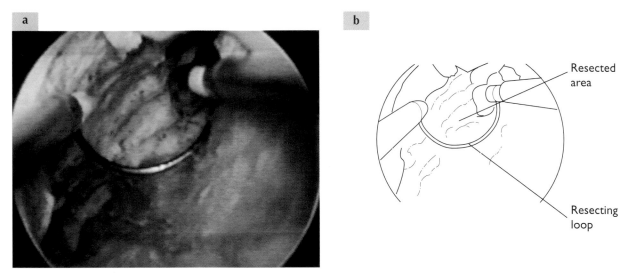

Figure 2.50 Loop resection of the posterior uterine wall: section of endometrium being resected.

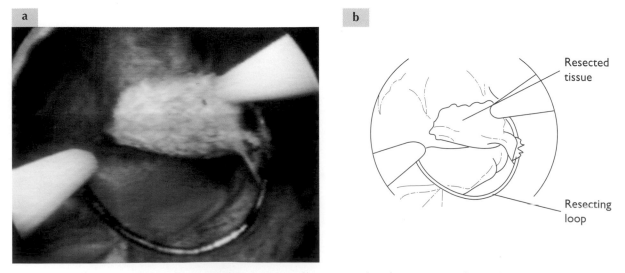

Figure 2.51 Loop resection of the posterior uterine wall: section of endometrium at the end of resection.

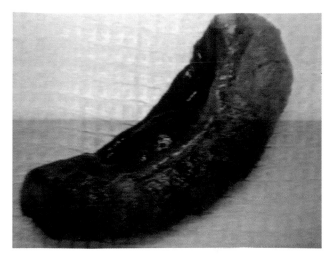

Figure 2.52 Section of endometrium after removal.

functional layer and the residual basal layer, unlike curettage, which withdraws only the functional layer and leaves the basal layer.

The thinner the mucosa, the easier the procedure will be. Medical preparation is necessary to thin the endometrium. This entails the use of either danazol for 4 weeks before the operation or a gonadotrophin releasing hormone analog such as depot leuprolide acetate for 2 months.

At surgery the first furrow is made on the posterior wall, starting close to the left tubal ostium. This first furrow usually makes it possible to determine the ideal depth of resection. The other furrows are made in the following sequence: posterior wall (left edge),

anterior wall (right edge), and posterior wall while moving the electric loop from the uterine fundus to the isthmus.

Electric wire loop resection
Electric wire loop resection (*Figs 2.49–2.55*) should begin at the left side of the posterior wall of the uterine cavity, starting at the left tubal orifice (*Figs 2.56 and 2.57*). Several adjacent grooves should be cut from the fundus towards the isthmus (*Fig. 2.58*), which must be left intact. This avoids the later formation of adhesions, which may impair subsequent examinations.

Hysteroscopic control provides a clear view of the border between the intracavity area where an endometrectomy has been performed – this area has a grainy yellowish surface – and the area near the isthmus untouched by the resectoscope – which has a well-vascularized, pink mucosa (*Fig. 2.59 a, b*).

Resection must not continue to the region of the horns, where the muscle wall is substantially thinner (*Fig. 2.60*). The liquid distension also creates a further thinning of the uterine wall in the region of the horns, increasing the risk of perforation. Here, electrocoagulation must be used.

The depth of the grooves can be checked by spacing them far enough to leave a strip of mucosa intact in between. This provides an indication of the original height of the uterine mucosa (*Figs 2.61 and 2.62; see Fig. 2.58*).

After electrosurgical endometrial ablation, a roller-ball electrode can be used to coagulate the entire

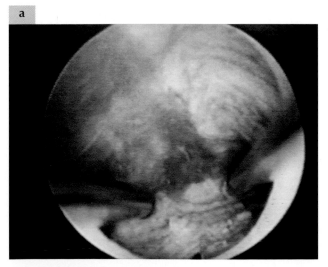

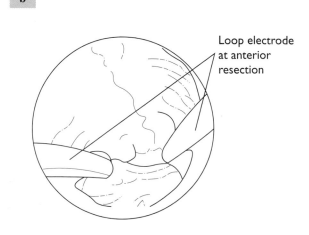

Loop electrode at anterior resection

Figure 2.53 Loop resection of the anterior uterine wall.

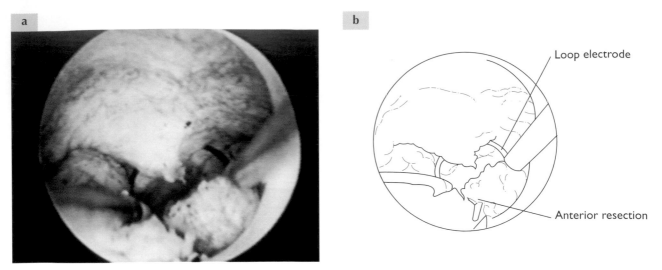

Figure 2.54 Loop resection of the anterior uterine wall: positioning of the loop electrode.

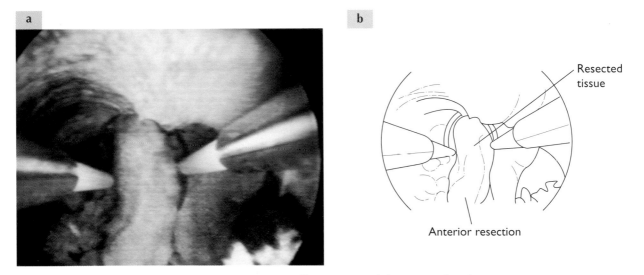

Figure 2.55 Loop resection of the anterior uterine wall: a portion of the resected endometrium.

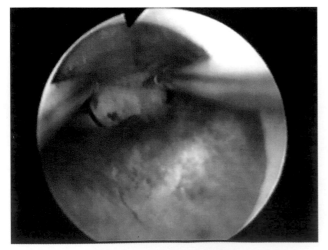

Figure 2.56 Endometrial resection: the first furrow is made on the posterior wall, beginning close to the left tubal ostium.

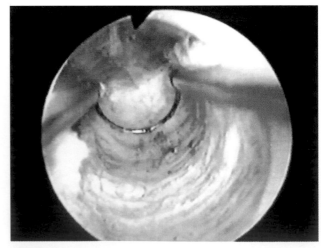

Figure 2.57 This first furrow usually determines the ideal depth.

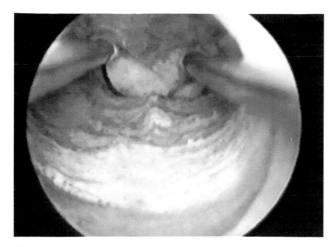

Figure 2.58 Several adjacent furrows should be cut from the fundus toward the isthmus. Furrow depth can be properly checked by spacing the furrows far enough to leave a strip of mucosa intact in between furrows. This will provide an indication of the original depth of the uterine mucosa.

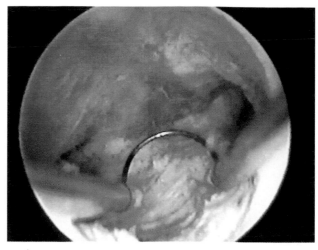

Figure 2.60 Resection of the endometrium on the anterior wall: resection must not continue to the region of the horns where the muscle wall is thinner.

a

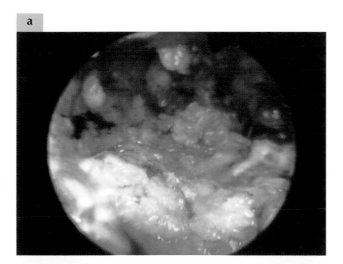

b

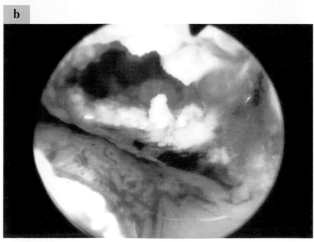

Figure 2.59 Hysteroscopic control provides a clear view of the border between the intracavity area where an endometrectomy was performed (grainy, yellowish surface), and the area near the isthmus that is untouched by the resectoscope (well-vascularized, pink mucosa).

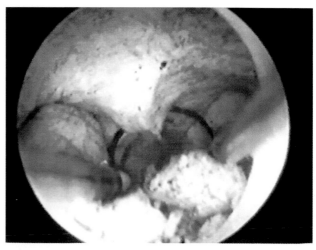

Figure 2.61 Resection of the endometrium on the right side.

Figure 2.62 The resectoscopic loop is cutting residual tissue between two furrows.

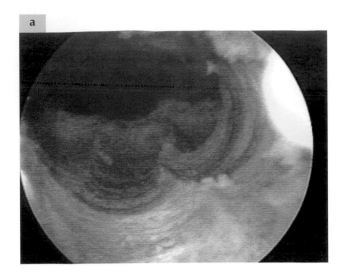

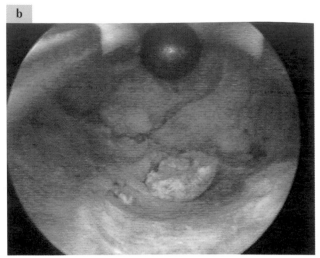

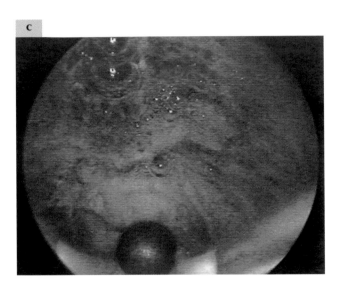

Figure 2.63 (a) View of the uterine cavity after an endometrial resection has been completed. After electrosurgical endometrial ablation, a roller-ball electrode can be used to coagulate the entire endometrial surface. (b) Roller-ball seen on the fundus and posterior wall. (c) Roller-ball on the anterior wall.

endometrial surface (*Fig. 2.63*). Less bleeding results when the two techniques are combined (*Fig. 2.64*).

Endometrial ablation using resection then coagulation is shown in *Figs 2.61–2.63*.

Resection has an advantage over laser photocoagulation and electrocoagulation in that it allows for histological study of mucosal cuttings, so endometrial cancer can be detected (*Fig. 2.52*).

The two techniques of endometrectomy by endoscopic resection or ablation with the Nd:YAG laser are very satisfactory for treating dysfunctional metrorrhagia. However, they require sufficient skill and experience for success. Rare but serious complications can occur:

- uterine perforation;

- metabolic problems caused by water overload hyponatremia related to glycine; and
- infection.

For this reason, another technique was proposed by Neuwirth in 1994 – thermocoagulation. Thermocoagulation uses a small heated balloon set up and inflated in the uterine cavity. This technique is as simple as that of the installation of an intrauterine device. Studies have shown that endometrial coagulation has the same effectiveness as that of endoscopic resection.

Nd:YAG laser photocoagulation
Nd:YAG laser photocoagulation (*Figs 2.65–2.69*) makes use of 600 μm diameter fibers and 55–80 W of power. Laser energy is transmitted by the application of the fiber to the mucosa (so-called

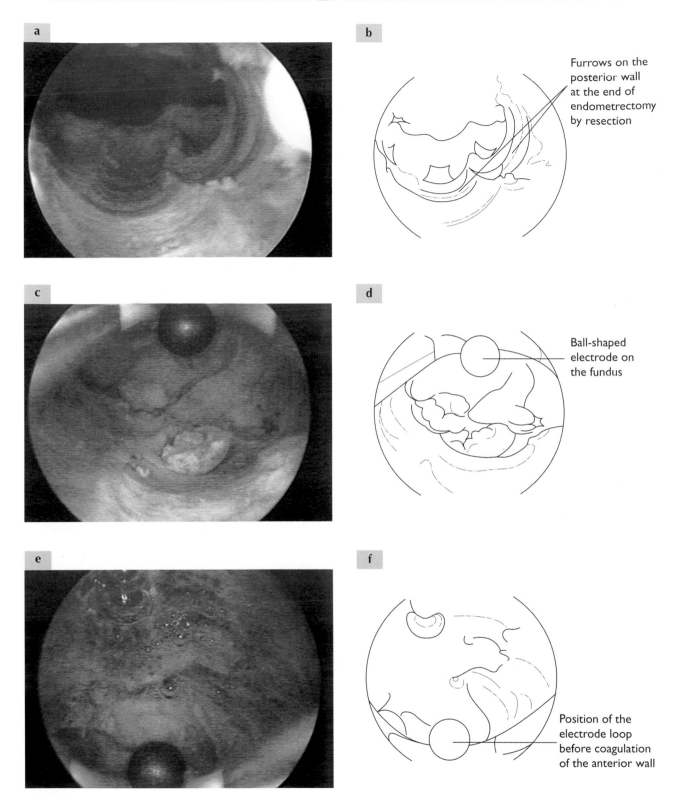

Figure 2.64 (a,b) View at the completion of an endometrial resection. (c,d) Electrocoagulation of the endometrium at the fundus and posterior wall of the uterus: the technique requires an unmodulated continuous sine wave, low voltage, current of 100–120W; it uses a 2 mm ball-shaped electrode that rotates freely on a spindle and cuts into the resected mucosa, causing it to become a caramel color. (e,f) The electrode loop is oriented for the coagulation of the anterior wall of the uterus.

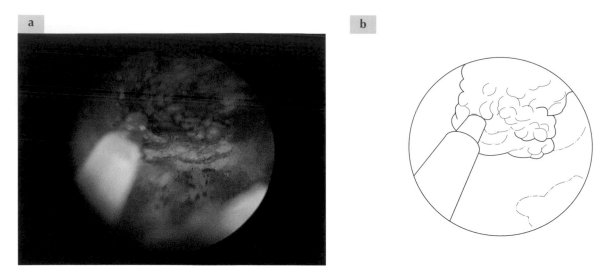

Figure 2.65 Endometrial ablation: start of procedure, photocoagulation of the right uterine horn.

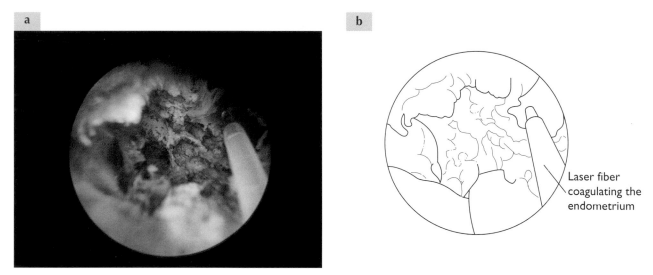

Laser fiber coagulating the endometrium

Figure 2.66 Endometrial ablation continued: photocoagulation of the fundus and left uterine horn.

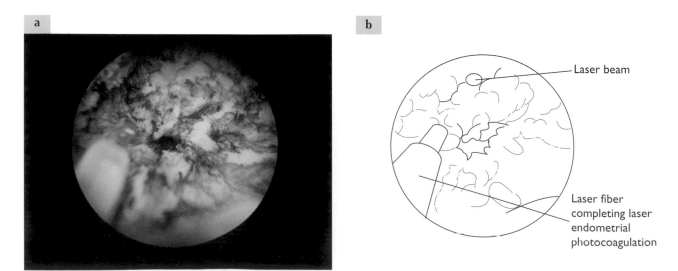

Laser beam

Laser fiber completing laser endometrial photocoagulation

Figure 2.67 Endometrial ablation continued: photocoagulation of the lateral walls.

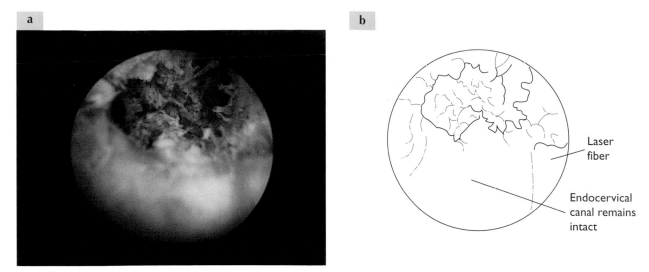

Figure 2.68 Endometrial ablation: end of procedure, the laser fiber is stopped at the isthmus, thereby leaving the endocervical canal intact.

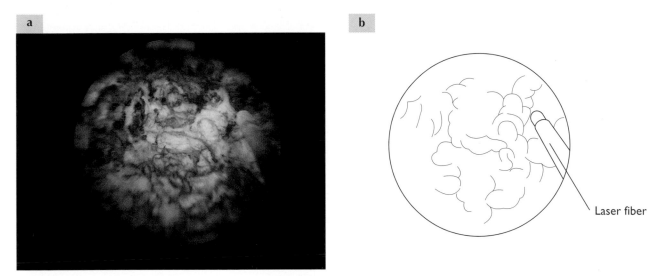

Figure 2.69 Endometrial ablation: end of procedure, the endometrial mucosa has been completely excised.

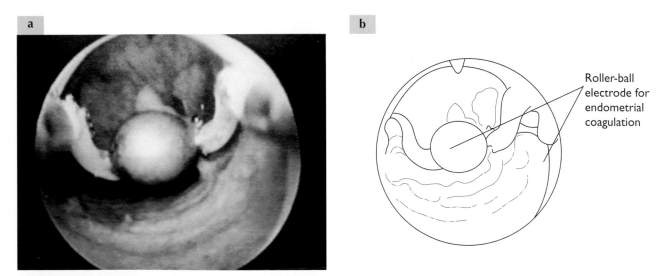

Figure 2.70 Roller-ball coagulation: start of procedure (left extremity of posterior uterine wall).

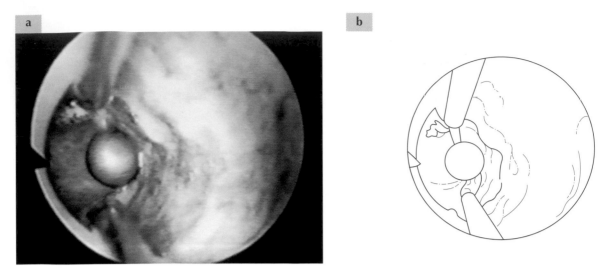

Figure 2.71 Roller-ball coagulation: procedure continues (right extremity of posterior uterine wall).

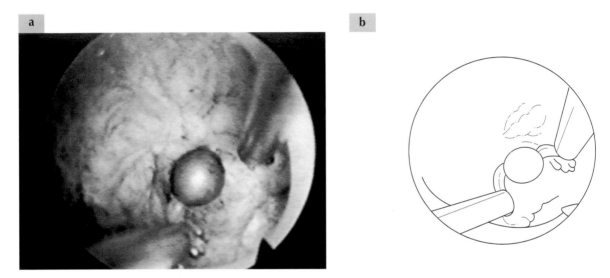

Figure 2.72 Roller-ball coagulation: procedure continues (anterior uterine wall).

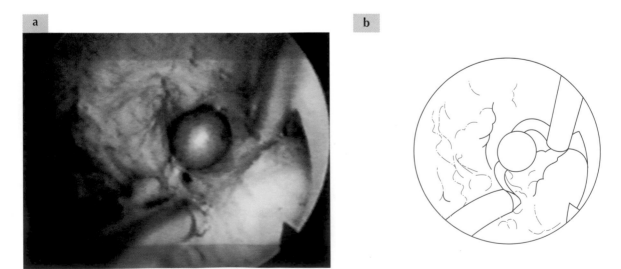

Figure 2.73 Roller-ball coagulation: procedure continues (anterior wall and fundus).

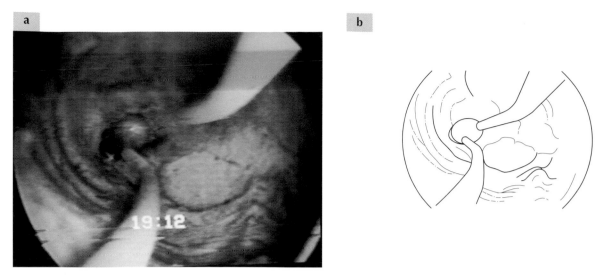

Figure 2.74 Roller-ball coagulation: procedure continues (right uterine horn).

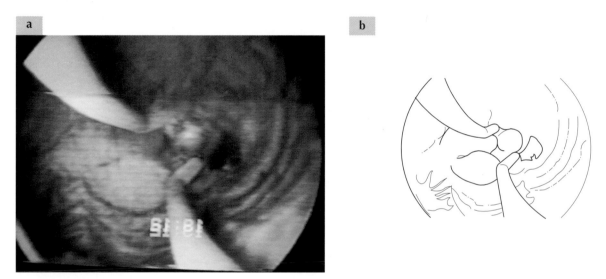

Figure 2.75 Roller-ball coagulation: procedure continues (left horn and fundus).

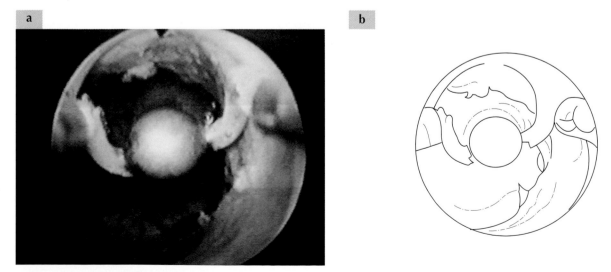

Figure 2.76 Roller-ball coagulation: end of procedure (coagulation is complete in the area of the uterine isthmus; the cervical canal is left intact to avoid the formation of adhesions at the isthmus that could inhibit postoperative surveillance.

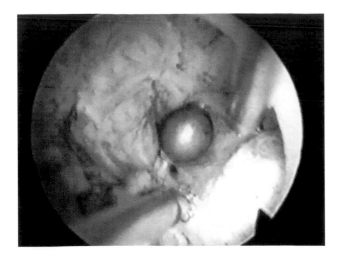

Figure 2.77 Electrocoagulation can be used to complete endometrial resection: roller-ball seen on the right uterine horn.

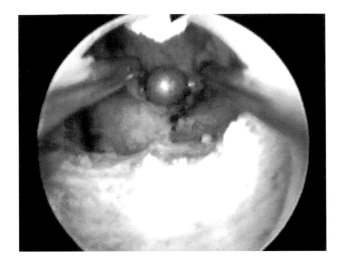

Figure 2.78 Electrocoagulation of the fundus.

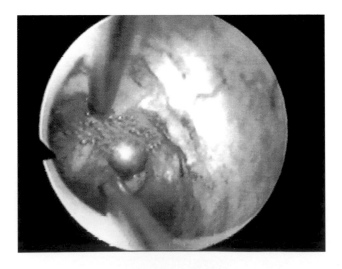

Figure 2.79 Electrocoagulation and hemostasis on the left side of the uterus.

technical contact or dragging). Alternatively, the core fiber laser can be fired 1–2 mm from the surface until the mucosa has been blanched (the so-called blanching technique).

Two months postoperatively, a control examination is necessary to ensure that the entire mucosa has been destroyed. The residual cavity takes on a yellow–white, grainy appearance, so any remaining islands of endometrium, which are pink and protruding, stand out very clearly.

Electrocoagulation of the endometrium
Electrocoagulation of the endometrium (*Figs 2.70–2.82*) makes use of a 2 mm ball-shaped

electrode or a broader roller-ball-shaped electrode rotating freely on a spindle. Coagulation (or modulated) current is within the range of 40 to 70 W; alternatively unmodulated (cutting) current of 100–120 W can be used. When the electrode cuts halfway into the mucosa causing it to become a 'caramel' color, the power is at the correct level.

Adenomyosis

Adenomyosis is an important pathology that can benefit from the technique of endometrectomy. It can be diverticular or interstitial. A third form of adenomyosis is the adenomyoma (*Figs 2.89 and 2.90*).

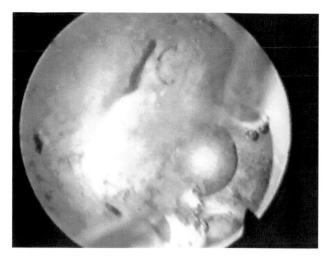

Figure 2.80 Electrocoagulation and hemostasis on the right side of the uterus: blood vessels are visible on the surface of the endometrium.

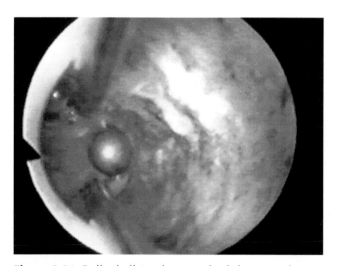

Figure 2.81 Roller-ball in place on the left uterine horn.

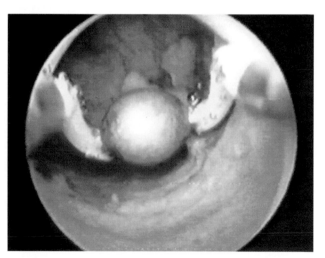

Figure 2.82 Electrocoagulation of the posterior uterine wall.

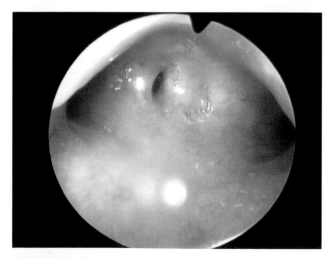

Figure 2.83 Diverticula of adenomyosis on the uterine fundus: the openings of the diverticula can be visualized provided that the mucosa is not too thick.

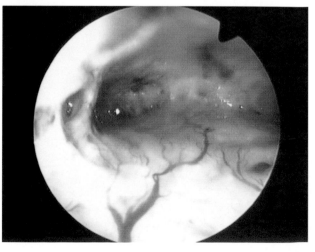

Figure 2.84 Diverticula of adenomyosis on the right side of the uterus. Numerous thin vessels are seen on the posterior wall.

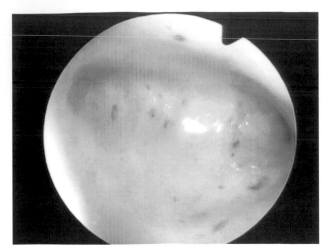

Figure 2.85 Diffuse interstitial adenomyosis, somewhat inhibited by preadministration of gonadotrophin releasing hormone agonists.

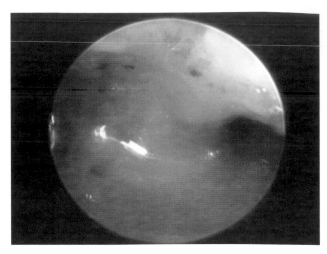

Figure 2.86 Interstitial adenomyosis on the uterine fundus: several small brownish spots.

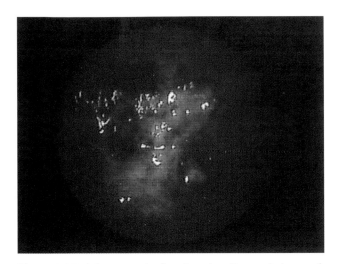

Figure 2.87 Adenomyosis showing the distorted shape of the muscular hypertrophy of the uterine base, giving a trabeculated appearance to the fundus.

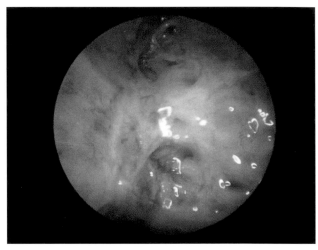

Figure 2.88 Adenomyosis in the uterine fundus: note the trabeculate appearance caused by hypertrophic muscular columns and diverticula.

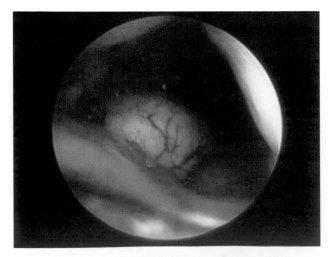

Figure 2.89 View of an adenomyoma that resembles a fibroma: the histological examination diagnosed the adenomyotic nature of this fibroma. The treatment is the same as that of a fibroma, namely endoscopic resection.

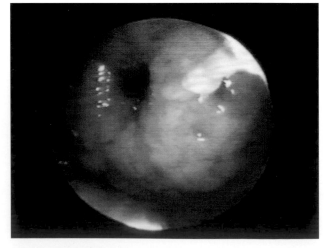

Figure 2.90 View of a voluminous adenomyoma with a diverticular orifice.

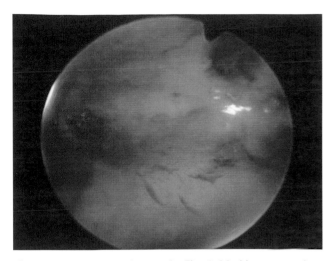

Figure 2.91 Same patient as in Fig. 2.89. Hysteroscopic control 2 months after resection of the adenomyoma.

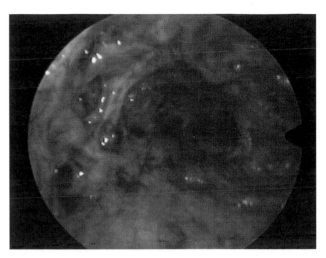

Figure 2.92 Endometrium following treatment with danazol. Danazol causes atrophy of the uterine mucosa, which has almost disappeared, thus revealing the muscle fiber bundles.

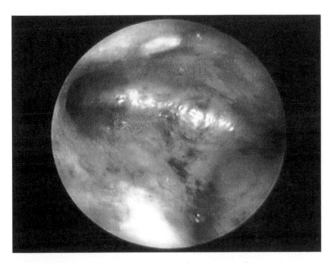

Figure 2.93 In a postmenopausal woman, the endometrium shows extensive atrophy, which accounts for abnormal bleeding.

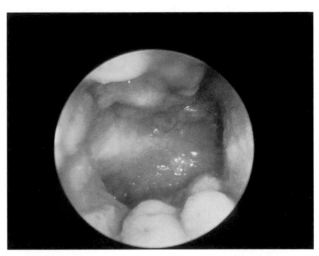

Figure 2.94 Generalized hyperplasia involving the whole mucosa and giving it a bumpy, indented appearance.

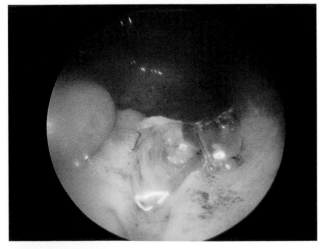

Figure 2.95 Hysteroscopic view of endometrial polypoid hyperplasia located on the posterior wall.

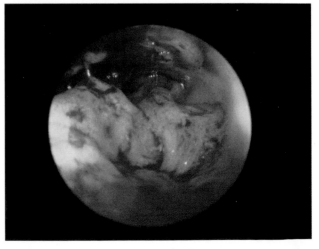

Figure 2.96 Widespread, typical adenomatous hyperplasia.

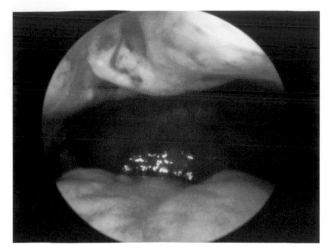

Figure 2.97 Typical generalized adenomatous hyperplasia.

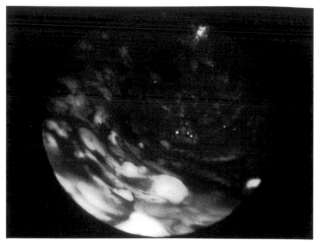

Figure 2.98 Atypical hyperplasia: pathology diagnosed endometrial adenocarcinoma.

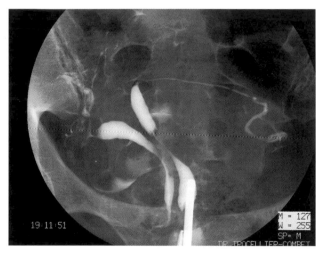

Figure 2.99 Hysterosalpingogram showing a broad-based septum going down to the cervix.

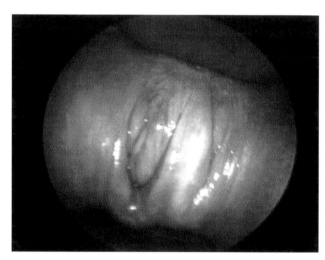

Figure 2.100 Same patient as in Fig. 2.99. View of the two cervices of the complete septate uterus.

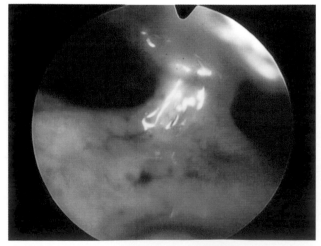

Figure 2.101 Subtotal septate uterus: the lower extremity of the septum is at the level of the isthmus.

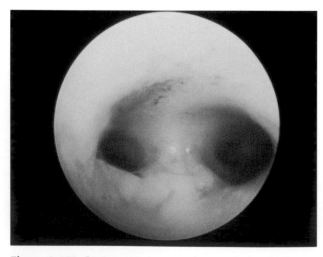

Figure 2.102 Septate uterus: partial corporeal septum.

Diverticular adenomyosis appears at hysteroscopy as small bluish or brownish spots or as small depressions of variable number and size within the mucosa (*Figs 2.83 and 2.84*). It is best to seek them immediately after menses. These lesions are most visible in postmenopausal women or in patients on therapy that causes atrophy of the endometrial mucosa.

Interstitial adenomyosis in fact represents islands of adenomyosis that have lost their direct connection with the surface of endometrium. When they are sufficiently close to the surface to be visible by transparency, they form bluish or maroon submucous spots (*Figs 2.85 and 2.86*).

Adenomyosis is often associated with muscular hypertrophy which results in a distortion of the uterine fundus (*Fig. 2.87*) where the columnar projections of the muscular bundles mix with the diverticula (*Fig. 2.88*).

The decision to use endometrectomy to treat adenomyosis is made primarily on the basis of endovaginal color Doppler ultrasound which allows for great selectivity in the indications. Thus, when the depth of invasion does not exceed one-third of the thickness of the myometrium, the preserving treatment is justified by proposing endometrectomy.

Adenomyoma (*Figs 2.89 and 2.90*) is a nodular formation that resembles a fibroma. Histological examination reveals a surface coating of cylindrocubic endometrial cells, and a very dense axis of chorion cells with endometrial glands in the medial and muscular layers.

Treatment is the same as for a fibroma – endoscopic resection (*Fig. 2.91*). Some patients are pretreated with danazol, gonadotrophin releasing hormone agonists or medroxyprogesterone, in order to cause the endometrium to undergo atrophy and so enhance its destruction. Danazol atrophies the uterine mucosa to the extent that it almost disappears, thus revealing the bundles of muscle fibers (*Fig. 2.92*). The appearance is very different from that of postmenopausal atrophy (*Fig. 2.93*).

Endometrial hyperplasia

Endometrial hyperplasia is another important pathology that can be treated with endometrectomy. It involves all or most of the mucosa, giving it a bumpy and indented appearance (*Fig. 2.94*). The narrowness of the cavity can prevent passage of the endoscope. The color of the mucosa is the same (gray–white) as during the second half of the menstrual cycle. The vasculature is abundant, fine, non-distended and varicose, as in endometrial

cancer. At times, the hyperplasia is focal to the point of resembling a polyp (*Fig. 2.95*).

Endometrial hyperplasia can be classified as:

- dystrophic (including simple hyperplasia and glandular–cystic hyperplasia); or
- dysplastic (including, in increasing order of severity, simple adenomatous hyperplasia (*Figs 2.96 and 2.97*), typical or active adenomatous hyperplasia, and atypical hyperplasia).

In the dystrophic hyperplasias, the stroma is rich in cells and the ratio of the glandular tube to the chorion is normal.

The dysplastic hyperplasias are characterized by an imbalance between the epithelium and the stroma: the epithelial cells proliferate to a greater or lesser degree, whereas the stroma regresses and becomes poorer in cells. The dysplastic hyperplasias cannot be identified by hysteroscopy and pathologists do not always agree on the interpretation of images. Therefore it is essential to rule out a small endometrial cancer before an endometrectomy is performed, since there may be particularly serious consequences if such a tumor is missed. A preoperative biopsy for histology must be taken at the time of the diagnostic hysteroscopy (*Fig. 2.98*).

Infertility

Uterine septa

Uterine septa are the consequence of an anomaly of development of the Müllerian ducts between the 11th and 14th weeks of fetal life, caused by the absence of resorption of the partition, which may be partial or total. It is the most common malformation and the most likely to result in loss of pregnancy. Associated urinary malformations are rare.

Hysteroscopic treatment can also be used in this condition. Hysterography shows a uterine cavity formed by two spindle-shaped parts and the uterine septum should be suspected if the fundal angle, caused by separation of the uterine horns, is less than 90° from each other. The V-shaped fundal defect is caused by a uterine septum (*Figs 2.99 and 2.100*).

According to the degree of the lack of resorption, the septate uterus can be:

- partially divided – subtotal (*Fig. 2.101*), corporeal (*Fig. 2.102*), or fundal; or
- completely divided, with or without a vaginal septum (*Fig. 2.103*).

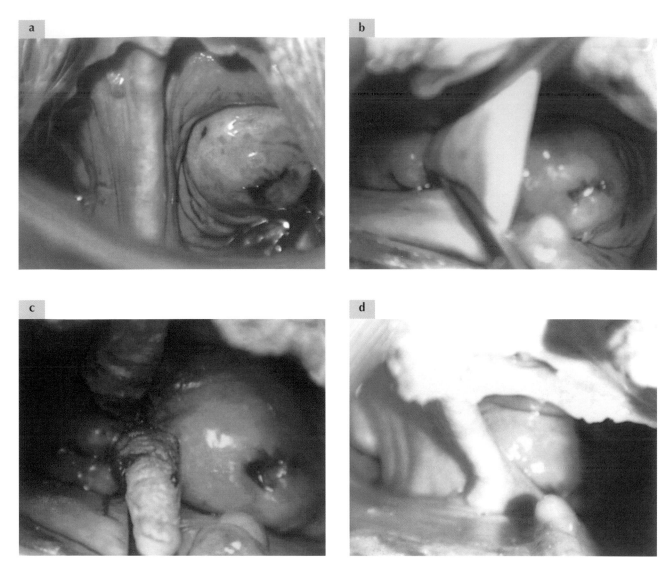

Figure 2.103 Section of a vaginal septum. (a,b) before sectioning. (c,d) after sectioning.

Ultrasound provides important information. It shows a normal uterus, externally, with a regular fundus and without median depression. There is no vesical projection between the two horns. Transverse sections show the malformation very well – an echogenic structure between the two cavities from where the aspect 'out of glasses' (*Fig. 2.104*).

Magnetic resonance imaging makes it possible to visualize the septum, which produces a fibrous-type signal in hyposignal T1 and T2, which measures the length of the fibrous septum. Laparoscopy enables a septate uterus to be distinguished from a bicornuate uterus – the septate uterus has a normal, broad serosal surface with a slight indentation in it (*Fig. 2.120c*).

Hysteroscopy shows the septum in the center (*see Fig. 2.101*) and the tubal orifices on each side in the optical axis (*Figs 2.105 and 2.106*), but it shows the thickness of the septum less well, especially at the base.

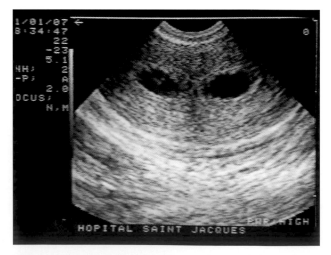

Figure 2.104 Preoperative ultrasound control. Note the 'binocular' appearance of the septum.

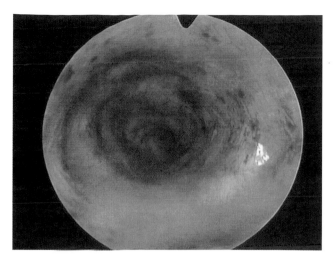

Figure 2.105 Right uterine horn in a uterus in which the two uterine horns are widely separated and each tubal ostium is clearly visible.

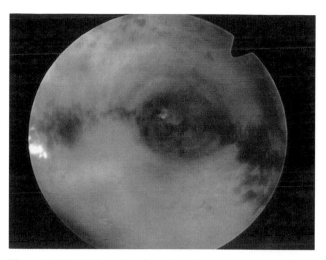

Figure 2.106 Left uterine horn in the same uterus as in Fig. 2.105.

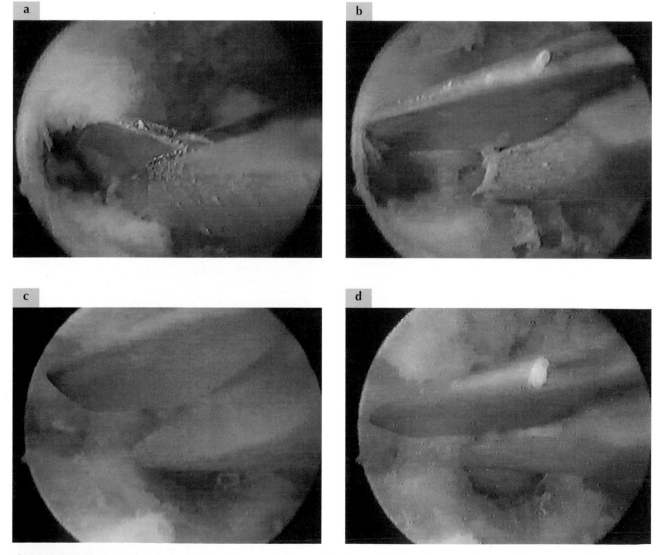

Figure 2.107 Four steps in a hysteroscopic penetration and scissors division of a complete uterine septum with septate cervix.

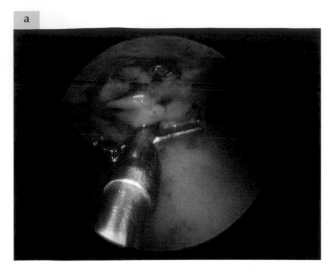

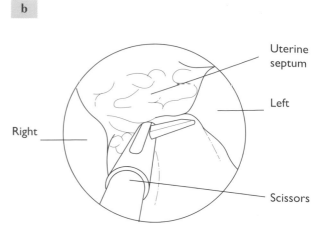

Figure 2.108 Uterine septum transection with scissors.

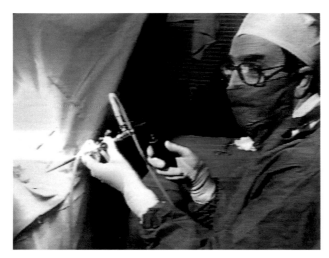

Figure 2.109 Installation of operative hysteroscope under video control.

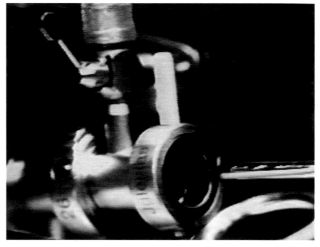

Figure 2.110 Insertion of the telescope into the operative channel of the hysteroscope.

Septal transection

Septal transection can be performed with scissors in a liquid or gaseous medium (*Figs 2.107 and 2.108*), with an Nd:YAG laser at a wavelength of 1.32 μm in a liquid medium (*Figs 2.109–2.112 and Fig. 1.31*) or with a straight resectoscope electrode in a liquid medium (*Fig. 2.113*). Laparoscopic and echographic control (using abdominal and endorectal probes) of the transection can provide a better and safer procedure in some cases (*Figs 2.114–2.116 and 2.117 see Fig. 2.104*).

The scissors technique has the advantage of simplicity. Scissors can be used if the septum is thin. The appearance of bleeding during the procedure indicates that the myometrium has been reached and that the sectioning is complete.

Septal section with a right loop of the resectoscope or the 'needle-tip electrode' of the Baggish hysteroscope has the disadvantage of causing more mucosal destruction. Therefore the use of the Nd:YAG laser is the technique of choice (*see Fig. 2.111*). The section is carried out upwards by successive sweeping movements (*Fig. 2.118*). It is bloodless and can be continued until a symmetrical uterine base has been achieved and the two tubal orifices can be seen

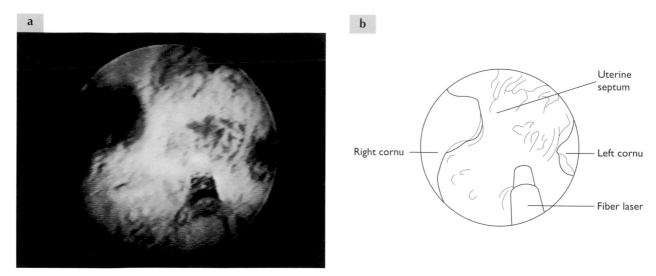

Figure 2.111 Transection of the septum using the Nd:YAG laser: start of procedure.

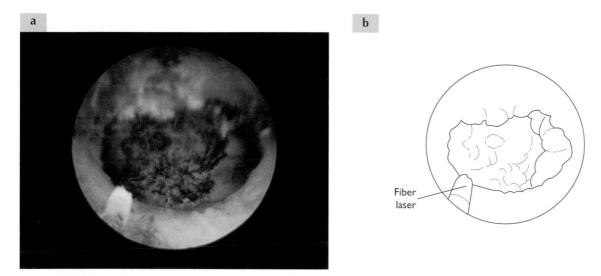

Figure 2.112 Septum transection using the Nd:YAG laser: appearance at the end of the procedure.

in the same field. Thanks to a per operative rectal echographic control per operational by rectal way, the section will be carried out until leaving a residual myometrial thickness of 12 mm (the wall of safety) (*see Figs 2.116 and 2.117*), so as not to weaken the uterine fundus (*see Fig. 2.112*).

A complete septum that extends to the cervix and the upper third of the vagina is treated by initially dividing the vaginal septum with scissors (of Mayo) (*see Fig. 2.103*) and then dividing the two cervices and the lower part of the uterine septum by slipping a blade on each side of the septum (*see Fig 2.107*).

A uterine coil is inserted to reduce adhesion formation. Two months later the remainder of the uterine septum is divided (*see Fig. 2.107*).

Hysteroscopy is performed 3 months after division of a uterine septum with scissors. When hysteroscopy reveals a residual upper portion of the septum, a second septal transection is necessary (*Fig. 2.119*).

Some gynecologists leave the cervical septum intact because it is believed that after its removal the patient is likely to develop an incompetent os

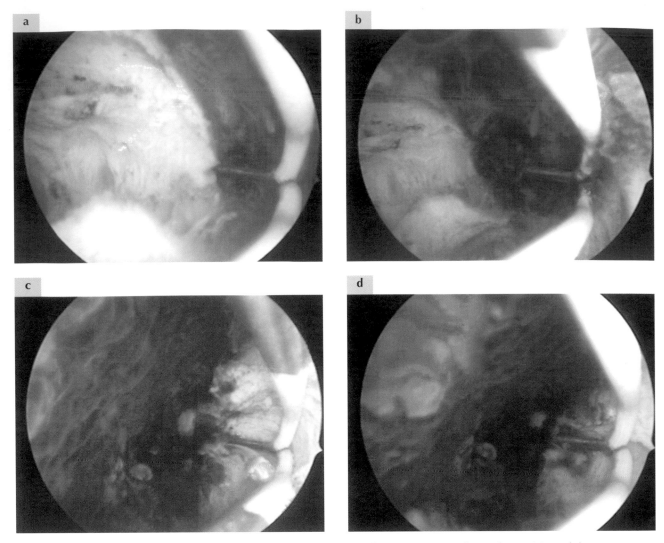

Figure 2.113 Electrosurgical cutting of a thick septum with a straight resectoscope electrode. Incision of the septum begins at the lower extremity on the left side (a,b) and on the right side (c,d), progressing upwards towards the fundus.

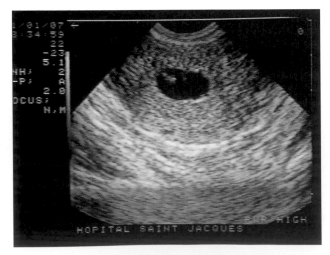

Figure 2.114 Ultrasound appearance of a uterine septum; note the rounded image below the septum.

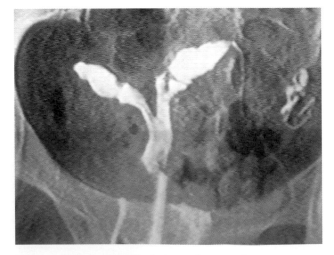

Figure 2.115 Radiological view of a partial septate uterus: hysterosalpingography shows a V-shaped fundus caused by the partial septum and widely separated uterine horns, the 2 semi uteri diverge but the fundal angle is less than 90°.

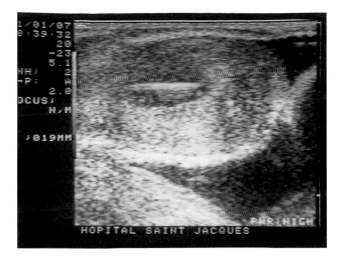

Figure 2.116 Intraoperative ultrasound to monitor progress of the resection: the thickness of remaining septum is 19 mm and the resection is insufficient.

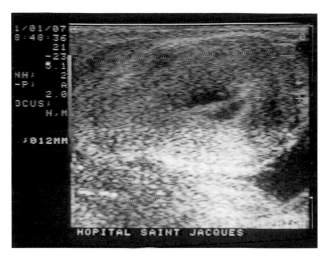

Figure 2.117 Ultrasound monitoring at the end of the procedure; 12 mm residual thickness 'security wall' remains, and the resection is satisfactory.

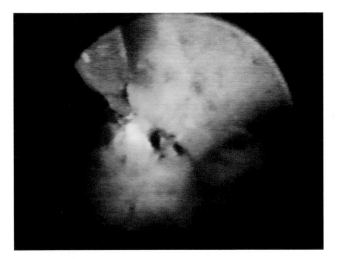

Figure 2.118 Septal transection with the Nd:YAG laser fiber: sectioning is performed upwards by successive cuttings.

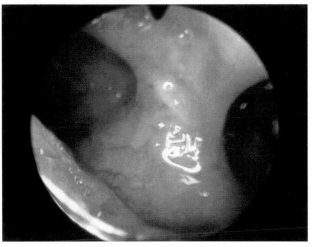

Figure 2.119 Hysteroscopic view 3 months after division of a corporeal septum with scissors. Note the residual upper portion of the septum. A second septal transection was necessary.

(Rock JA and Jones HW Jr). After the intervention, antibiotics are given for 5 days, and sequential hormone treatment (estrogen–progesterone) is given for 2 months. Hysteroscopic control is needed when the the coil is removed. However, because of generally good results, postoperative medications are generally no longer needed.

Clinical case 1

A 25-year-old patient with a separation of the cervix, uterus and vagina.

Diagnosis

1. Hysterography reveals a completely divided uterus. The septum is complete and two separate, almost symmetrical cavities are formed (*Fig. 2.120*)

The septate uterus was confirmed by laparoscopy; in this case, the uterus was not bicornuate. The septate uterus has a normal serosal surface, with a slight indentation and without vesicorectal division.

A hyperechogenic median septum was identified by pelvic ultrasound.

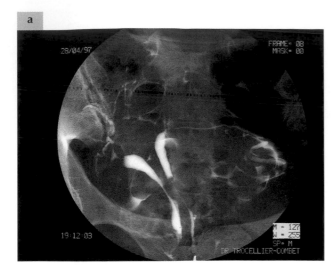

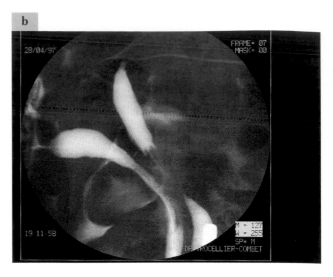

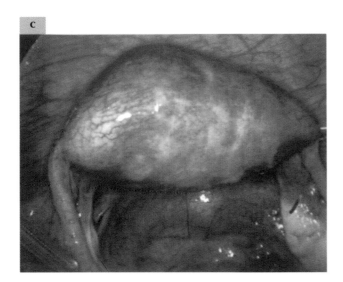

Figure 2.120 (a,b) Radiological views of the complete septate uterus. (c) Laparoscopic view showing a normal serosal surface of the septate uterus, a whitish area of tissue is visible in the median transverse diameter that indicates the fundal origin of the septum.

2. Clinical examination with the aid of a vaginal speculum can visualize the double cervix (*Fig. 2.121*). Hysteroscopy is used to assess the size and extent of the septum.

3. Hysteroscopy reveals part of the right uterine hemicavity and the right lateral wall of the very thick total uterine septum (*Fig. 2.122*).

Operative procedure

4. The procedure begins with sectioning of the vaginal septum held taut by two tenacula. Each of the two cervices is reclined laterally using a Pozzi forceps (*Fig. 2.123*).

5. A 5 mm metal bougie (or Hegar dilator) is positioned in the right cervical os, and a 4 mm metal bougie is positioned in the left cervical os.

After sectioning the intracervical septum, a larger, 8 mm bougie can be positioned in the (now single) cervical os (*Fig. 2.125 g,h*).

6. Intraoperative views of the total uterine septum using glycine solution (1.5%) (*Fig. 2.126*).

7. Intraoperative views of the use of the straight electrode to cut the left edge and then the right edge of the septum. Septal transection rather than resection is the procedure of choice (*Fig. 2.127*).

8. One month after resection of the septum, the appearance of the single cervix is satisfactory (*Fig. 2.128*).

9. Six months after the procedure, there remains a small residual septum in the uterine fundus, which draws together the uterine walls in the proximity of the fundus (*Fig. 2.129*).

A further procedure will be performed on the remaining septum at a later date.

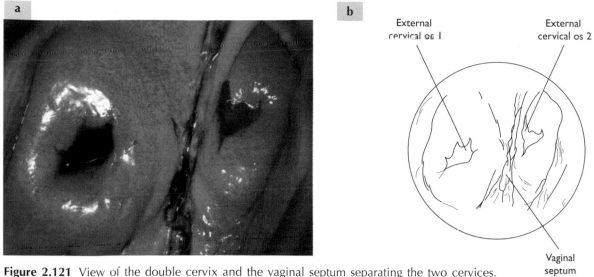

Figure 2.121 View of the double cervix and the vaginal septum separating the two cervices.

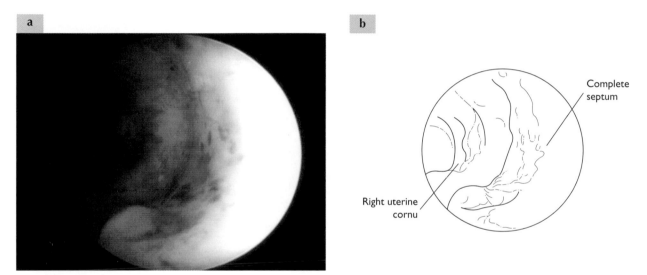

Figure 2.122 Hysteroscopic view of part of the right uterine hemicavity and the right lateral wall of the very thick total uterine septum.

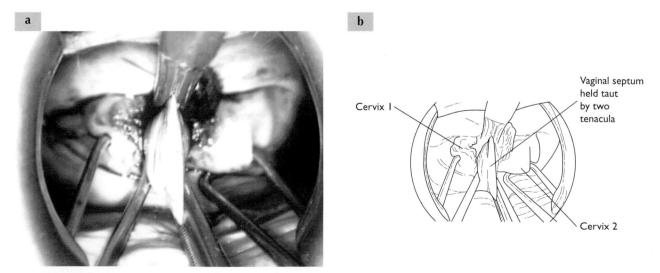

Figure 2.123 Sectioning of the vaginal septum.

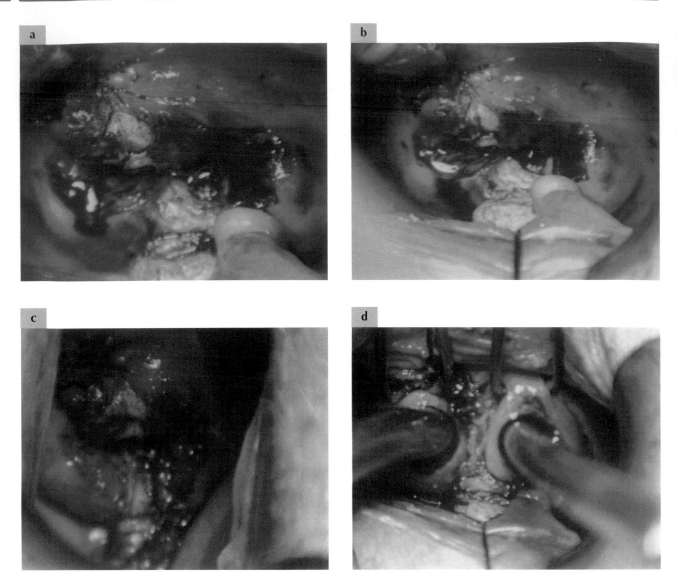

Figure 2.124 After section of the vaginal septum, the two cervices are catheterized with metallic probes (a,b,d) and the lower part of the uterine septum is resected. Aspect of the single cervix after resection of a total septum (c).

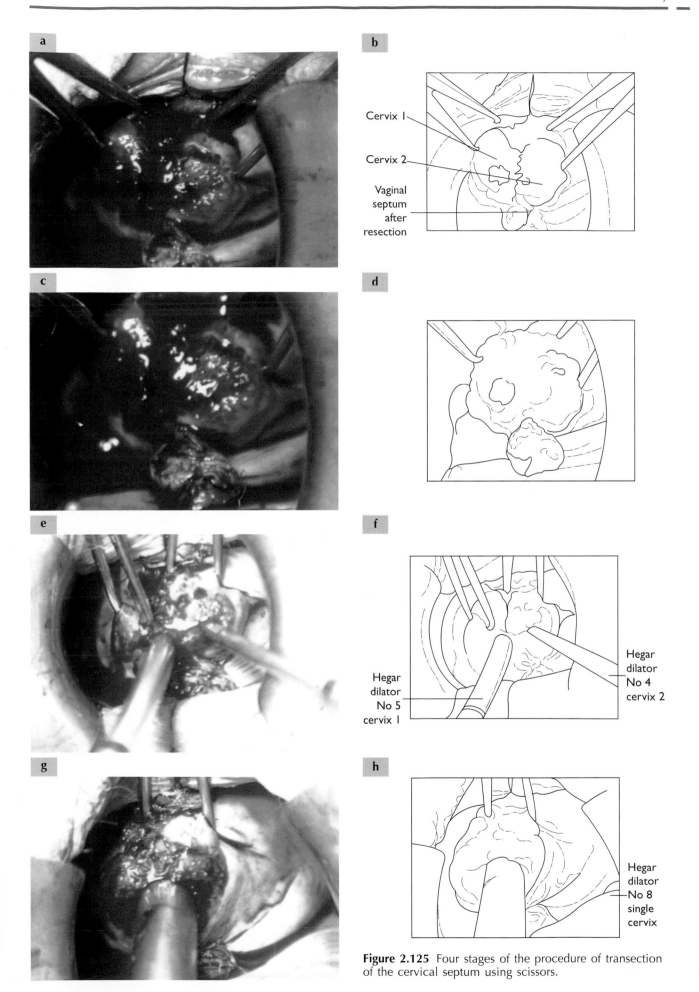

Figure 2.125 Four stages of the procedure of transection of the cervical septum using scissors.

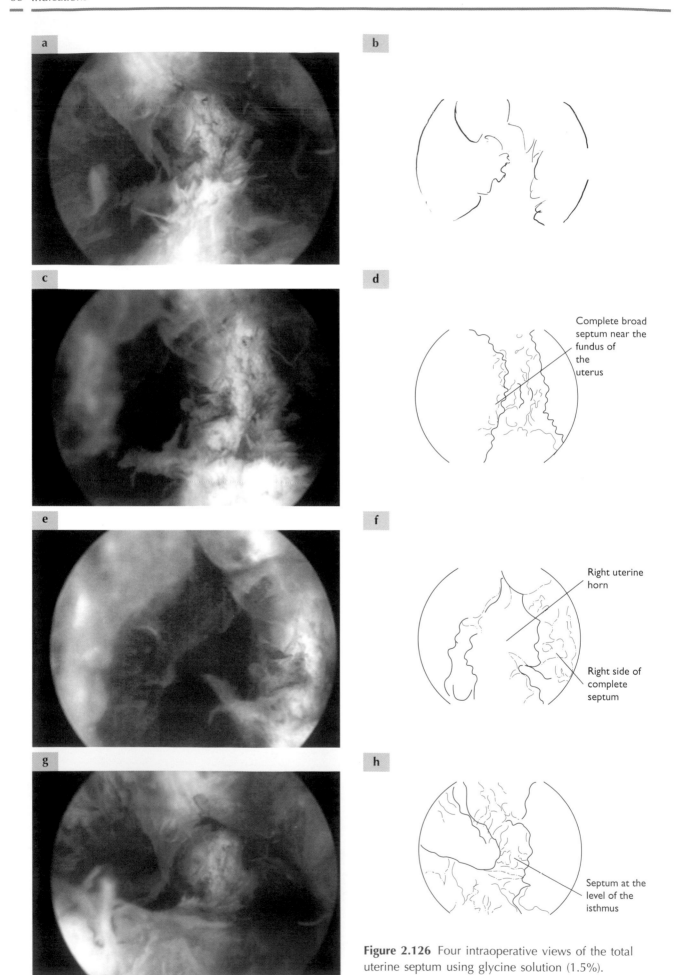

Figure 2.126 Four intraoperative views of the total uterine septum using glycine solution (1.5%).

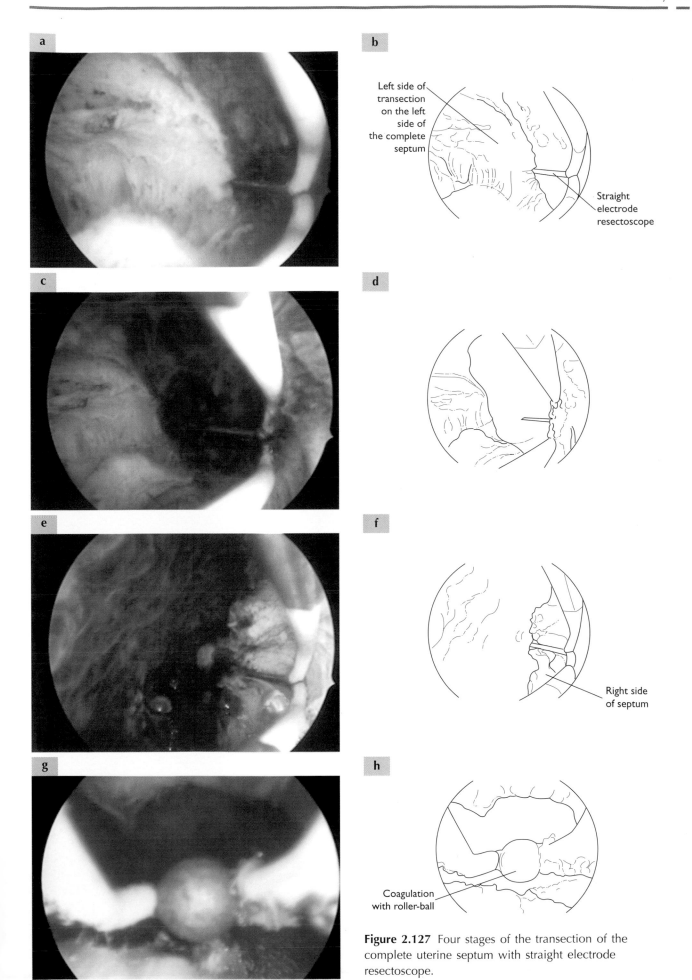

Figure 2.127 Four stages of the transection of the complete uterine septum with straight electrode resectoscope.

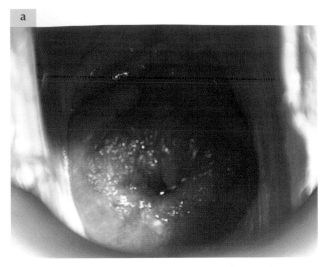

Figure 2.128 Satisfactory appearance of the single cervix.

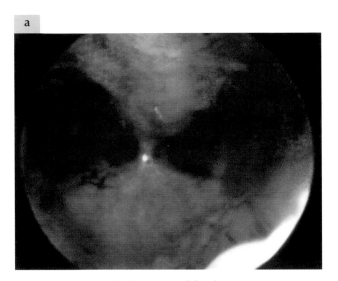

Figure 2.129 Residual septum of fundus.

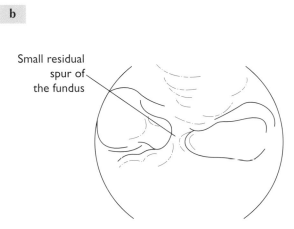

Small residual spur of the fundus

Clinical case 2

1. Mrs. M. (aged 42 years) suffered three sponta-
    neous abortions. Hysteroscopy reveals a partial
    septate uterus (*Fig. 2.130*). Hystero-
    salpingography disclosed a V-shaped fundus
    caused by a partial septum and widely separated
    uterine horns.

Laparoscopic findings 1 month later were of a
normal uterine serosal surface. The septum was
resected using the scissors on a Baggish operative
hysteroscope.

Pregnancy followed and, 1 year later the patient
delivered a healthy baby at 8 months' gestation.

2. Hysteroscopic examination 18 months after
    delivery revealed a well-delineated residual
    septum in the uterine fundus, which accounted
    for the premature birth (*Fig. 2.131*).

Congenital anomalies

Uterine malformations may occur in women who
were exposed to diethylstilbestrol *in utero*. In the
majority of cases, hysterography shows a T-shaped
uterus with a hypoplastic cavity and a constricting
band in the middle of the uterine cavity (*Fig.
2.132*).

The hypoplastic endometrial cavity as well as
disturbances of ovarian function (abnormal ovarian

a

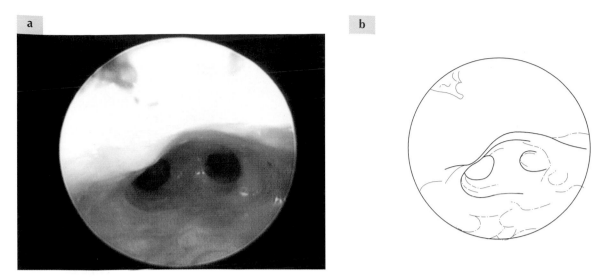

Figure 2.130 Hysteroscopic appearance of a uterine partial septum of a 42-year-old woman.

a

b

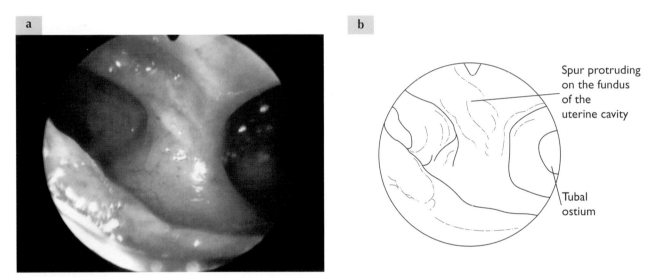

Spur protruding
on the fundus
of the
uterine cavity

Tubal
ostium

Figure 2.131 Hysteroscopic result 2 years after septum transection, showing the existence of a well-delineated residual septum in the uterine fundus.

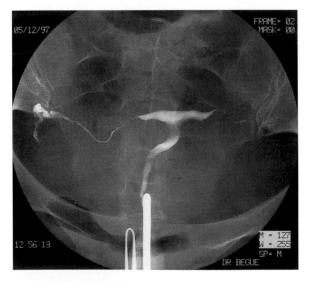

Figure 2.132 Hysterosalpingogram showing a T-shaped uterus in a diethylstilbestrol-exposed girl, before treatment.

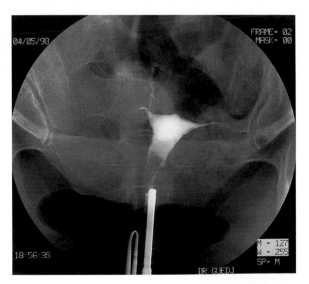

Figure 2.133 Hysterosalpingogram of the same patient as in Fig 2.132 after treatment. Three years later pregnancy followed and the patient delivered by cesarean section a healthy baby at 8 months' gestation.

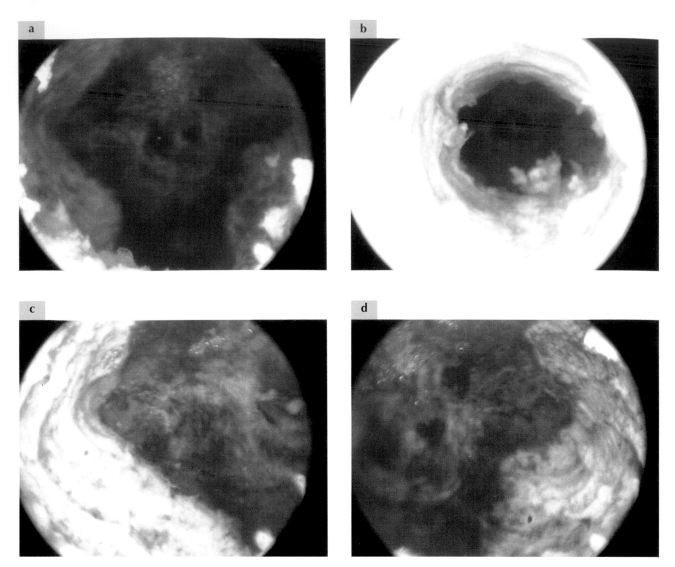

Figure 2.134 Enlargement of a T-shaped uterus with a right electric loop. (a,b) Before operation: hysteroscopic view of the hypoplastic uterus. (c) After incision of the narrow side walls: view of the right side wall. (d) View of the left side wall after incision.

follicular maturation) can cause reduced fertility. The hypoplasia also affects the external morphology of the uterus and endometrial surface with a particularly fine endometrium. There may also be obstetrical repercussions such as extrauterine pregnancies, miscarriages, and premature births.

Operative hysteroscopy can be used for treatment. After a hysterographic diagnosis, an echographic assessment is necessary to ascertain the size of the uterus and the thickness of the uterine walls.

The purpose of hysteroscopic intervention is to enlarge the uterine cavity using an Nd:YAG laser or an electrode (*Fig. 2.134 a,b*). Sectioning begins at the top from the right angle formed by the two branches

of the 'T' and continues on each side until a uterine cavity of normal shape is obtained. A coil is inserted and left for 2 months. Estrogens are given during this time.

The anatomical results of this type of operation are excellent (*Figs 2.133 and 2.134 c,d*). However, future obstetric care must be in a specialized center well equipped to deal with two possible complications: uterine rupture and uterine hemorrhage.

Asherman's syndrome (lysis of adhesions)

Intrauterine adhesions may be defined as the joining of the walls of the uterus. They may be total, when

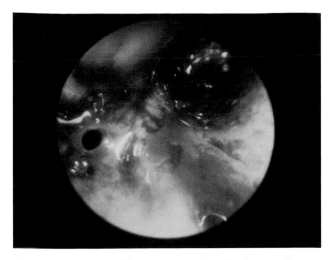

Figure 2.135 Large fibrous corporeal adhesion sparing the two uterine horns.

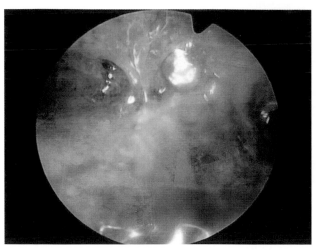

Figure 2.136 Column-shaped synechiae in the fundus of the uterus.

they cover the whole of the uterine cavity, or partial, when they affect only one part of the uterine cavity or cervix. In 1948 and 1950, Asherman defined two entities of intrauterine lesions according to hysterographic criteria:

- traumatic intrauterine adhesions and
- stenosis of the internal cervical os.

Hysteroscopy allows the diagnosis of the synechiae, specifies their location and extent and classifies them as fibrous or sclerous. Hysterography is indicated in the event of complex adhesions or of a total synechiae of the isthmus (See Appendix, Figs A58 & A59).

Some intrauterine adhesions are recent and not very wide and can be easily broken by the simple pressure of the hysteroscope. Older synechiae are thicker and more resistant. They are made of connective tissue or of a combination of collagen bundles and muscles fibers. Their surface is white and not very vascular.

Three types of synechiae are observed:

- multiple and wide adhesions, which create a thick screen in the uterine cavity and more or less completely mask the uterine base (*Fig. 2.135*);
- columnar adhesions, which are localized adhesions that form a column of varying thickness that joins the two walls of the uterine cavity (*Fig. 2.140*); the adhesion is broader at the points of fixation than in the middle, giving it

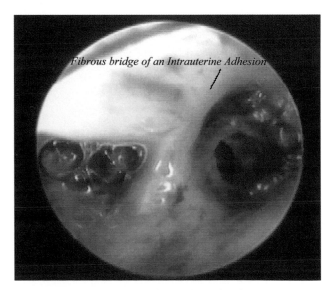

Figure 2.137 Corporeal column-shaped adhesion with an hour-glass appearance: the broad fibrous bridge separates the two horns simulating a septum.

an hour-glass shape (*Fig. 2.137*); these adhesions are usually on an anteroposterior axis but they can also be oblique; and
- marginal adhesions, which are crescent-shaped and are made up of a system of multiple fibers; they are whitish in appearance and their preferred site is at the edges of the uterine cavity (*Fig. 2.140*), although they can also be anterior, central, oblique or in the uterine fundus (*Figs 2.138, 2.139 and 2.140*).

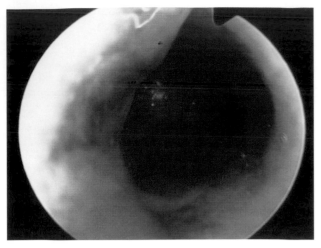

Figure 2.138 Crescent-shaped marginal adhesion on the right uterine side before division by hysteroscopic pressure.

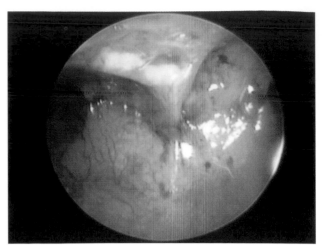

Figure 2.139 Crescent-shaped adhesion in the fundus.

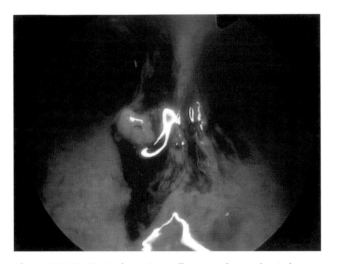

Figure 2.140 Central uterine adhesion above the isthmus, partitioning the uterine cavity.

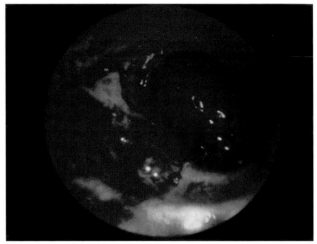

Figure 2.141 Marginal adhesion after division.

Procedure

Treatment of the adhesions is difficult; moreover, it must be as perfect as possible at the first operation because recurrences of badly operated synechiae can be impossible to treat. The ideal is to restore the normal anatomy of the uterine cavity, for which there are three techniques of operative hysteroscopy:

- rupture of the synechiae by hysteroscopic pressure, used for recent, mucous or poorly organized synechiae (*Figs 2.138 and 2.141*);
- resection of synechial scar tissue with the electric loop of a resector, which runs the risk of partial destruction of the endometrium; and
- simple section in the good plan of the joining, with scissors, which is the technique of choice for organized and resistant synechiae (*Fig. 2.142*).

Sectioning with endoscopic scissors preserves tissues integrity. It has the advantages of simple intrumentation and rapid implementation. It is ideal for central synechiae and complex synechiae (*Figs 2.140, 2.142 and 2.143*).

Indeed, with the needle electrode, the current section of the synechiae is used in monopolar mode and not in bipolar mode as with the resectoscope. The needle electrode can also be used as an instrument of coagulation in monopolar mode. It is effective but it is not without risk: accidents of intestinal burns have been described even in the absence of any uterine perforation.

Nd:YAG laser treatment at wavelength 1.32 μm is the treatment of choice. The laser beam is absorbed well by clear tissues, it cuts close to that of the laser with CO_2. It is used for complex synechiae, together with scissors.

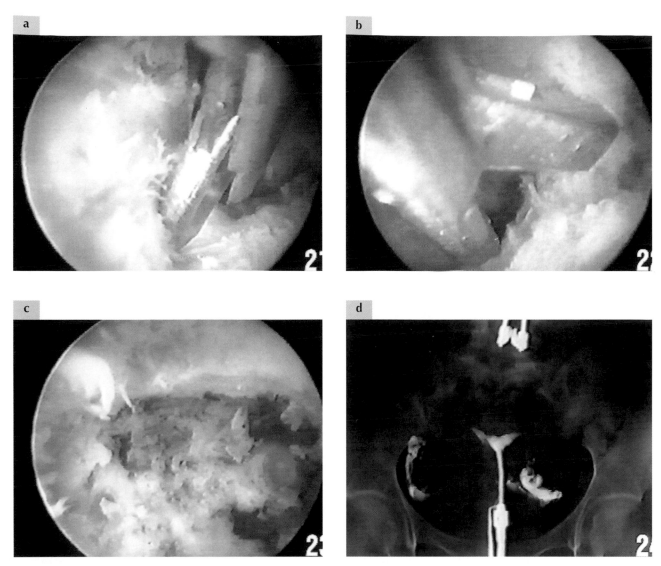

Figure 2.142 Division of thick, extensive intrauterine adhesion (a,b), completed procedure (c) and postoperative hysterosalpingogram (d).

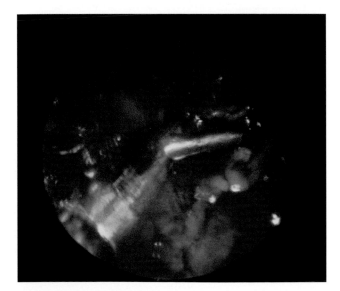

Figure 2.143 Lysing of corporeal adhesion using endoscopic scissors.

Echographic guidance for operative procedures is useful for following the progression of the cut compared with the uterine base and the uterine horns.

Recurrence of adhesions is prevented by installing a coil or a Kehr drain that has been cut to the dimensions of the reconstituted cavity.

Sequential estrogen treatment is given for 2 months to promote epithelial regeneration.

Tubal cannulation

The insertion of a catheter into the fallopian tube is relatively easy. The purpose of catheterization is:

- to treat obstacles at the uterotubal junction; and
- to transfer zygotes or gametes as a part of fertility treatment (ZIFT, zygote intrafallopian transfer).

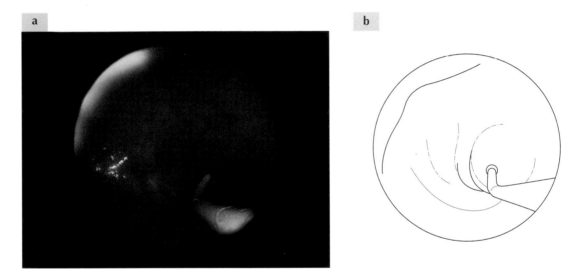

Figure 2.144 Tubal cannulation: catheter approaching the tubal ostium.

Left tubal opening

Tubal catheter approaching tubal opening

Figure 2.145 Tubal cannulation: catheter within the ostium.

Anatomy

The fallopian tubes prolong the uterine horns towards the ipsilateral ovary. The fallopian tube travels transversely at first and then passes superiorly alongside the ovary to end at the posterior edge of the ovary. The precise anatomy varies according to the position of the uterus and the presence of tubal pathology.

The fallopian tube measures 12–15 cm in length and has four segments:

- the tubal ostium, measuring 0.8–1 mm;
- the intramural portion, measuring 1.5 cm with a lumen of 0.5 mm diameter, it is sinuous in shape, making catheterization difficult;
- the isthmic portion, measuring 3–4 cm, with a lumen of 1 mm diameter; and

- the ampullar portion, measuring 7–8 cm, with a lumen of 5–8 mm diameter.

Methods of tubal cannulation

Catheterization under hysteroscopic control is indicated for patients with a history of infertility whose hysterosalpingography shows a proximal unilateral or bilateral tubal obstruction. A catheter containing a very fine metal wire is introduced into the tubal lumen. This wire can be conveyed by a rigid hysteroscope provided with an Albarran bridge to direct it towards the tubal ostium. Distension of the cavity is achieved with glycine solution. The catheter is pushed through the tubal ostium (*Fig. 2.144*) and pushed back and forth to find the direction of the intramural portion (*Fig. 2.145*). This

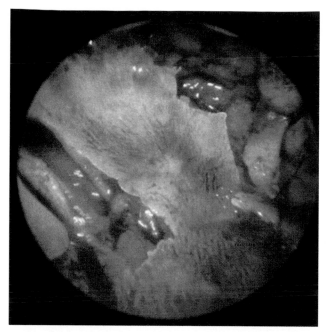

Figure 2.146 Osseous metaplasia: visualization of numerous irregular bony chips.

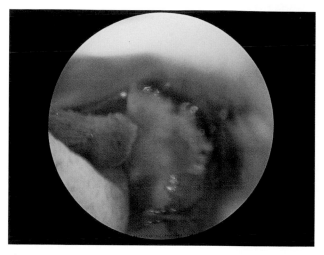

Figure 2.147 Endometrial ossification with spicules of bone.

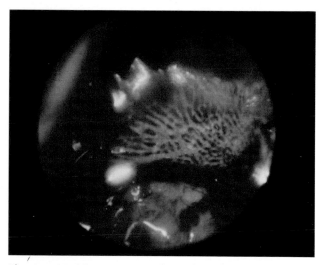

Figure 2.148 Osseous metaplasia: bony fragments with a 'crabshell' appearance digging into the mucosa.

allows the removal of obstructions from the proximal portions of the tube. Once the catheter is in place, the metal guide is withdrawn and replaced if necessary by an optical fiber. A fibroscope may be useful because of its flexibility.

Obstructions may have an organic origin, or may be the after-effect of a tubal infection or be caused by a spasm or be due to a purely mucous synechia. The easiest pathologies to treat are thin intratubal adherences or the fibrinous bridges that occur after spontaneous miscarriage.

The optimal time for this type of exploration is in preovulary stage.

Osseous metaplasia

Osseous metaplasia is a less common condition than those described above. It is characterized by the presence of irregular osseous remnants in the uterine cavity. They may appear like flat bones or long bones (*Fig. 2.146*).

The pathogenesis seems to be related to the retention of osteogenic elements after a miscarriage (often a late miscarriage). One also supports the hypothesis of the possible formation of an osseous metaplasia. Osseous metaplasia is generally discovered during investigations for a secondary sterility or an unexplained metrorrhagia; sometimes it is found because of relatively minor problems such as pelvic pain.

Diagnosis

Hysterography may show unusual images with vague, irregular lesions at variable sites and without clear limits. Some of these images may look like an adenocarcinoma, but the age of the patient usually mitigates against this diagnosis.

Ultrasound gives images that are difficult to interpret and may raise the possibility of a retained fragment of a uterine coil.

Hysteroscopy makes the diagnosis easy – whitish chips of irregular form are seen, and these chips feel hard when they come into contact with the hysteroscope (*Figs 2.147 and 2.148*).

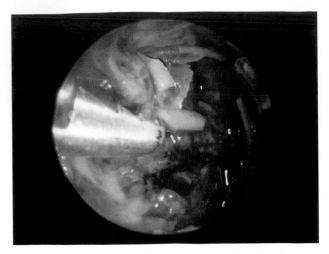

Figure 2.149 Removal of endometrial ossification by forceps under visual control.

Treatment

Ablation of the sheets of bony tissue is always delicate, since the lesions are embedded in the wall. The osseous elements are withdrawn one by one under visual monitoring using a grasping forceps slipped into the operative channel of the hysteroscope (*Figs 2.149 and 2.150*). The procedure is repeated as often as necessary until the uterine cavity is completely empty. A hysteroscopic evaluation is performed 1 month later to check for residual fragments which can be the cause of recurrence.

Oncology

Hyperplasia of the endometrium

Hyperplasia (or hypertrophy) of the endometrium is defined by the development and the thickening of one or more elements of the endometrial mucosa – the chorion, the glands, or the cylindrical epithelium. Hyperplasia may occur with or without atypia.

Endometrial hyperplasia without atypia

Simple hyperplasia
Simple hyperplasia is characterized by the harmonious increase in glandular epithelium and normal stroma. The surface is corrugated and may contain pseudopolyps. The vessels, which are not very abundant, are normal (*see Fig. 2.95*).

Glandular–cystic hyperplasia
Glandular–cystic hyperplasia presents with small glandular cysts surrounded by small vessels.

Adenomatous hyperplasia
Adenomatous hyperplasia causes imbalance between the epithelium, which proliferates, and the stroma which is poor in cells. The vascularization is regular. Adenomatous hyperplasia is at the border of atypical adenomatous hyperplasia; distinction between the two is only by histology (*see Figs 2.96 and 2.97*).

Endometrial hyperplasia with atypia

Hyperplasia with mild atypia
There is a small increase in glands compared with the stroma, and there is cytonuclear atypia.

Hyperplasia with moderate atypia
There is a clear increase in glandular tissue compared with the stroma, and there is an increase in the cellular size and the nucleus.

a

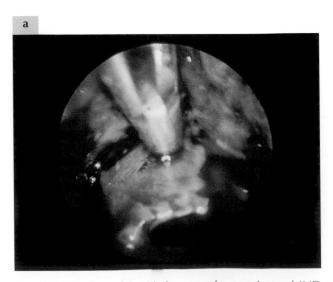

b

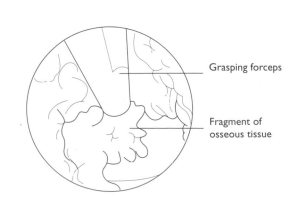

Grasping forceps

Fragment of osseous tissue

Figure 2.150 Removal with forceps of a translocated IUD under visual control.

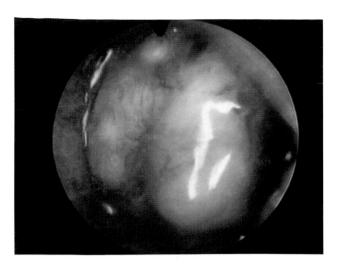

Figure 2.151 This polypoid form of cancer is less common; it can resemble an ordinary polyp with a multilobular appearance.

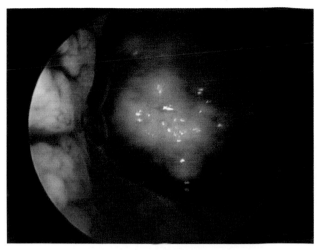

Figure 2.152 Multilobular pedunculated submucous myoma that resembles a mixed malignant tumor.

Hyperplasia with severe atypia
There are glandular buddings with papillary invaginations and nuclear stratifications, and severe cellular atypia (*see Fig. 2.98*).

Differentiation between types of endometrial hyperplasia
Generally these lesions must be differentiated by histology, since the macroscopic aspect seen with hysteroscopy does not allow a reliable diagnosis. Any decision to treat endometrial hyperplasia by endometrectomy that is made on the basis of hysteroscopic findings must therefore be backed up by an endometrial biopsy under visual monitoring (with or without a paracervical block) in order not to miss a developing cancer.

Endometrial carcinoma

The diagnosis of cancer of the endometrium can be strongly suspected after hysterosalpingography. It is difficult to confirm the diagnosis with ultrasound.

Hysteroscopy is the most useful examination because it can be combined with targeted biopsies and because it can delineate the extent of the disease and establish whether the isthmus and cervical channel are affected. Hysteroscopy can establish the cause of metrorrhagia in the perimenopausal period – budding, friable, hemorrhagic lesions or less serious pathologies, such as hypervascularized polyps or thick, heterogeneous mucous formation with irregular hypervascularization (*see Appendix, Figs A68–A70*).

Differential diagnoses that must be made before operative hysteroscopy

Cancer versus hyperplasia
Hysteroscopy has a significant role to play in the diagnosis and evaluation of endometrial cancer. However, as noted above, histological examination is required to avoid performing an endometrectomy for a lesions that is in fact an adenocarcinoma.

Cancer versus polyp
Rarely an endometrial cancer can have the shape of a large, multilobular polyp (*Fig. 2.151*).

Cancer versus fibroma
Some fibromas have a rather irregular, multilobular appearance and can look like a mixed malignant tumor (*Fig. 2.152*).

Uterine sarcoma
A special case is endometrial carcinosarcoma (*Fig. 2.153*). These mixed malignant tumors are being seen more and more often. They account for 1–3% of uterine cancers. Because of their seriousness, they cannot be ignored.

There are two cancerous components – adenocarcinoma of the endometrium and sarcomatous degeneration of the stroma (including leiomyosarcoma, fibrosarcoma or undifferentiated sarcoma). In some cases, the sarcomatous degeneration is heterologous and includes rhabdomyoblasts (rhabdomyosarcoma),

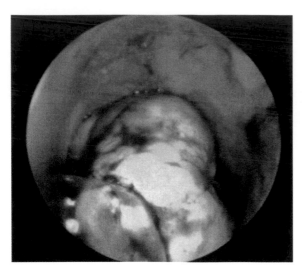

Figure 2.153 Carcinosarcoma of the fundus and posterior wall of the uterus (75% mortality 5 years after hysterectomy).

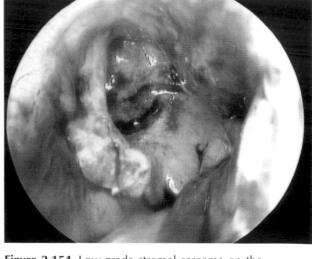

Figure 2.154 Low-grade stromal sarcoma on the posterior wall and right uterine horn (80% long-term survival after hysterectomy).

malignant-looking cartilage (chondrosarcoma), or bone (osteosarcoma).

Two forms of uterine sarcoma that present different hysteroscopic appearances and are of different seriousness are shown in *Figs 2.153 and 2.154*. *Figure 2.154* shows a stromal sarcoma that appears as necrosed irregular polyps that are traversed by numerous, often slack vessels. Histological examination showed a proliferation of endometrial stroma without any visible tube. *Figure 2.153* shows a carcinosarcoma on the uterine fundus and posterior wall. Macroscopic diagnosis is difficult, and the lesion can appear like a fibroma on hysterography and hysteroscopy. The danger in lesions such as this is to perform an endoscopic resection of what is in fact a serious malignant tumor.

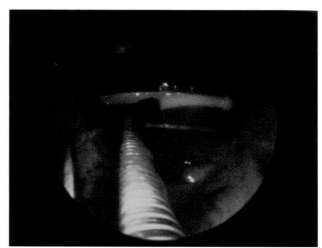

Figure 2.155 An IUD with thread that has ascended into the uterine cavity.

Other conditions

Lost intrauterine devices

When the thread of an intrauterine device (IUD) is not visible at the external cervical os, endoscopy can confirm the proper placement of the IUD (*Figs 2.155 and 2.156*) and facilitate grasping of the thread and removal of the IUD with forceps (*see Fig. 2.150 and 2.158*), unless the uterine cavity is empty. If the cavity is empty the IUD has either been expelled or has perforated the uterus, and a laparoscopy is necessary. Less frequently the IUD has incompletely penetrated the uterine wall, so part of it is visible by laparoscopy and the rest via a vaginal approach. The easiest point of access needs to be determined; it is generally that which affords free access to the IUD fragment.

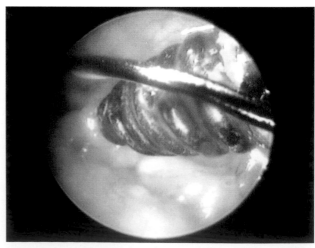

Figure 2.156 The IUD string is ascended and the device is embedded into mucosa.

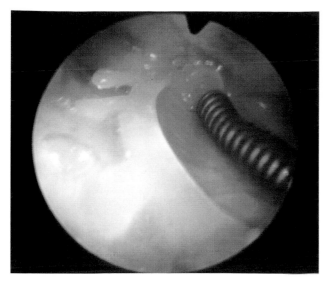

Figure 2.157 Displaced IUD on the left uterine horn.

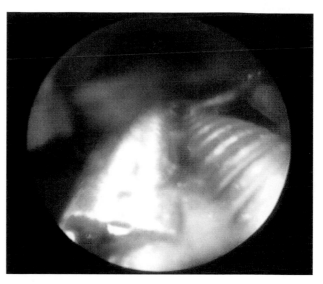

Figure 2.158 Retrieval of a lost IUD by forceps under visual control.

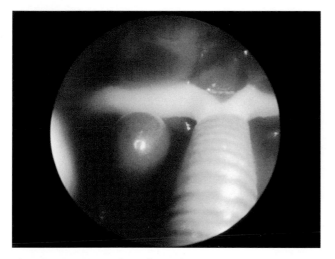

Figure 2.159 An IUD and a polyp.

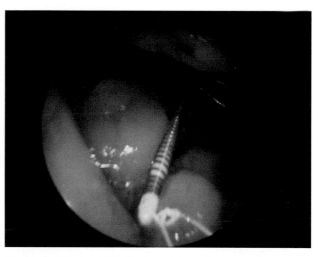

Figure 2.160 An IUD displaced by submucous myomas.

Misplaced or displaced IUD

More often, the IUD remains in the correct plane but shifts away from the ideal axis (*Fig. 2.157*). In this case, when retraction is attempted, the thread usually breaks or works free from the IUD, in which case ablation under visual control is required (Fig. 2.158).

Other IUD problems

IUD and menometrorrhagia

Hitherto undiagnosed organic lesions may be at the root of metrorraghia. Hysteroscopy can reveal a latent polyp associated with an IUD (*Fig. 2.159*), a fibroma (*Fig. 2.160*), or hyperplasia (*Fig. 2.161*). Operative hysteroscopy is necessary, with resection of the lesion and removal of the IUD.

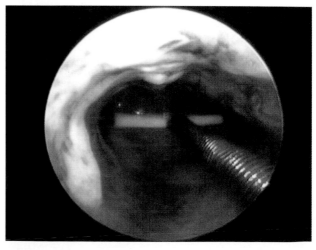

Figure 2.161 A T-shaped IUD and focal hyperplasia.

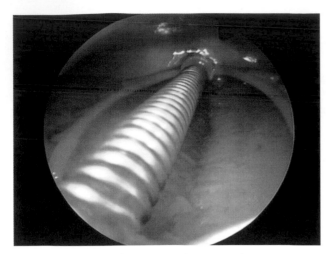

Figure 2.162 Properly positioned IUD: in this case, no intrauterine lesion is present, and so dysfunctional bleeding can be diagnosed.

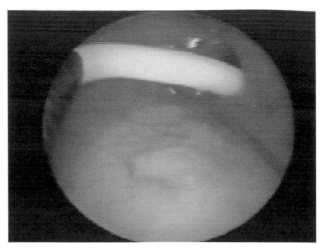

Figure 2.163 Displaced IUD: the arms of the 'T' are ranged obliquely and embedded into the mucosa.

If no organic lesion is visible, the metrorraghia is functional (*Fig. 2.162*).

IUD and pelvic pain

Sometimes an IUD is found lying perpendicular to the plane of the uterine cavity with the arms of the IUD penetrating into the uterine wall, causing pain and metrorraghia (*Fig. 2.163*).

IUD and pregnancy

The IUD usually lies on top of a gestational sac in a pregnant uterus, and the removal of the IUD is performed under visual control without risk of interruption of the pregnancy (*Fig. 2.164*).

Other foreign bodies

Other foreign bodies in the uterus include suture threads and laminaria used for dilatation before a curettage. Hysteroscopy is very useful in determining the location, direction, shape and size of remnants of the laminaria. It is easy to grasp the pieces of laminaria and remove them with a Kelly forceps.

Tubal sterilization

Hysteroscopic sterilization is theoretically a very good technique, the hysteroscope allowing an easy visualization of the tubal ostium. However, in practice, laparoscopy remains the only practical and reliable method.

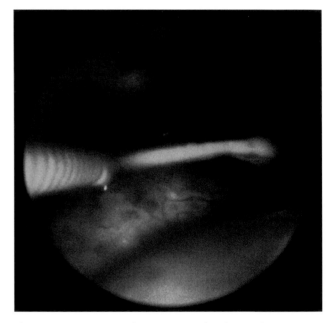

Figure 2.164 IUD and pregnancy: the device lies on top of a gestational sac; it can be removed under visual control without risk of interrupting the pregnancy.

Five techniques of hysteroscopic sterilization are possible:

* tubal electrocoagulation or cryocoagulation – this technique is of little interest because of the rate of significant failures (nearly 50%) and of the many serious complications (e.g. extrauterine pregnancy, intestinal burns).
* injection of sclerosing substances – various chemical agents are used; including quinacrine and methyl cyanoacrylate; however, the failure rates are still too high, at 20%.

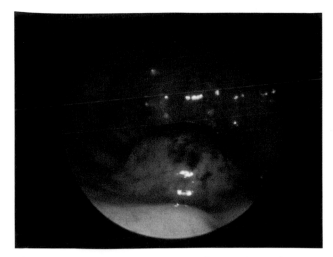

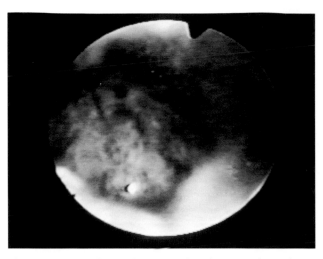

Figure 2.165 Hysteroscopic view of an embryo after 5 weeks of amenorrhea: the ovum pushes the mucosa into a hemispherical bulge, the surface of which is smooth and highly vascularized.

Figure 2.166 Embryo after 9 weeks of amenorrhea: the ovum is located on the posterior wall.

- sterilization using the Nd:YAG laser – the fiber is introduced 1 cm into the interstitial portion of the tube, where it acts by contact with the tubal mucosa with a power of 80 W; this technique is easy to perform but the results are not always long-lasting.
- hysteroscopic tubal occlusion with silicone rubber plugs – silicone rubber plugs are directly formed in place to block the oviducts; the success rate is approximately 85%; failures are generally due to migration or expulsion of the plug or a defective plug; and
- installation of intratubal devices – this process is tempting because it allows reversibility (at least theoretically); several kinds of devices made of nylon or silicone, with or without hooks, are used; for sterilization by silicone plugs, a pump is used to inject silicone. Intratubal devices or microcoils are presently being clinically evaluated.

However, all these techniques are far from achieving the results of the laparoscopic methods.

Hysteroscopy during pregnancy

Hysteroscopy with uterine distension by CO_2 is absolutely contraindicated during early pregnancy. It is important to recognize early pregnancy – the ovum pushes the mucosa up into a hemispherical bulge, the surface of which is smooth and highly vascularized (*Fig. 2.165*).

The only endoscopic technique that can be performed during pregnancy is contact hysteroscopy. The contact hysteroscope is a single instrument because it does not require any distension of the uterine cavity, which could cause a termination of the pregnancy. Because of its hard core of optical glass mineral, this instrument collects the ambient light and transmits it through an optical guide. It allows satisfactory visualization, even in the presence of mucus, by light contact with the epithelium or the structure to be looked at.

The contact hysteroscope has multiple applications:

- embryoscopy – the examination of the pregnancy is done between 4 and 10 weeks (*Fig. 2.166*); the development and anatomical differentiation of the embryo, can be followed;
- control of the uterine cavity after termination of pregnancy by induced abortion or spontaneous miscarriage;
- evaluation of postpartum metrorrhagia – membranous fragments or residual placental tissue can be seen in the area of the uterine horns, and a directed curettage can then be performed to stop the hemorrhage quickly;
- amnioscopy – the hysteroscope is gently guided into the cervix and light contact is made on the amnion; this examination is performed in an atraumatic way between 28 weeks and full-term; the color of the amniotic liquid can be observed in order to evaluate the fetal risk;
- diagnosis of a hydatiform mole – characteristic molar vesicles appear as blue edematous chorionic villi; and
- chorionic biopsy – early antenatal chromosomal diagnosis can be made by first-trimester chorionic biopsy with a 4 mm or 6 mm contact hysteroscope.

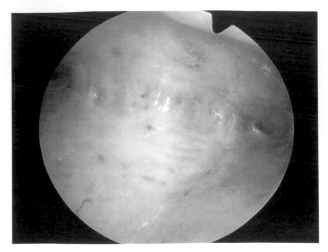

Figure 2.167 Uterine cavity after 2 months of treatment with luproreline or a gonadotrophin releasing hormone agonist. The extensive endometrial surface shows atrophy, the endometrium is flat and smooth all over with no visible glandular ostia. Many blood vessels are clearly discernible.

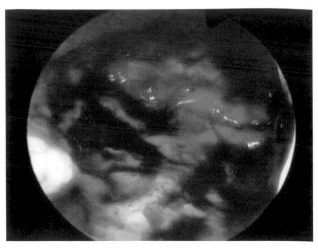

Figure 2.168 Endometrial cavity 4 weeks following endometrial ablation.

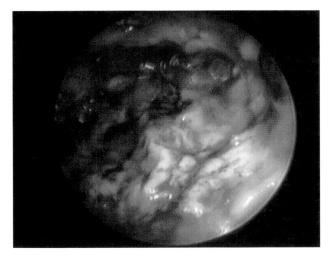

Figure 2.169 Endometrial cavity 3 months after endometrial ablation with a resectoscope: the cavity has a shrunken, yellow–white appearance.

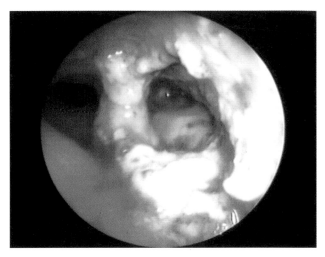

Figure 2.170 Hysteroscopic view 1 year after endometrial ablation: the endocervical canal alone is accessible to the hysteroscope. The uterine cavity has become a narrow passage.

Atrophy of the endometrium after gonadotrophin releasing hormone analogs

Gonadotrophin-releasing hormone agonists are largely used to decrease the thickness of the endometrium before an endometrectomy (*Fig. 2.167*) (e.g. to decrease the size of fibroma before resection). The effect of these agents on the hypothalamic–pituitary axis is due to a significant but reversible reduction in estrogen levels, resulting in a marked atrophy of the endometrium. This endometrium preparation makes it possible to shorten the operative time appreciably.

The histopathological effects of leuprolide acetate is a reduction in the glandular and vascular elements.

Residual endometrium after endometrial ablation

A hysteroscopy is performed 2 months after an endometrectomy. This examination is particularly significant because it makes it possible to see whether the totality of the mucous membrane has indeed been destroyed (*Fig. 2.168*). The residual uterine cavity has a shrunken, white–yellow appearance (*Fig. 2.169*). Any small island of mucosa that has not been destroyed appears clearly as a projecting, pink zone. It can then be destroyed by laser. One year after the endometrectomy, the cavity is more narrowed and admits just the hysteroscope, giving a 'finger-shaped' image on hysterography (*Fig. 2.170*).

3 Hysteroscopic results: preoperative and postoperative views

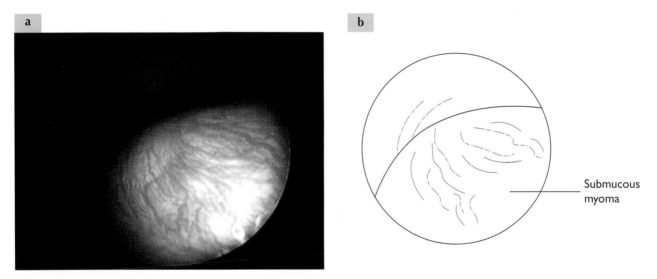

Figure 3.1 Submucosal myoma on the anterior uterine wall before resection.

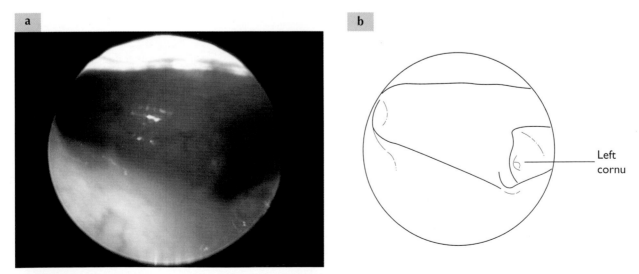

Figure 3.2 Four months after resection: very good result.

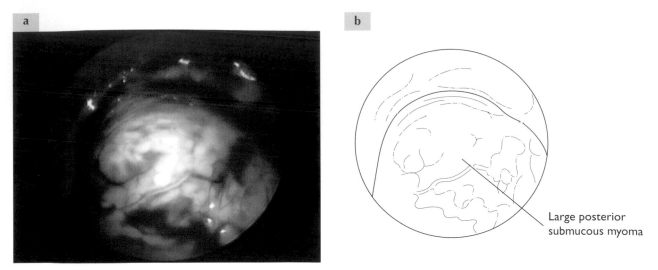

Figure 3.3 A large submucosal myoma in the fundus and the posterior wall.

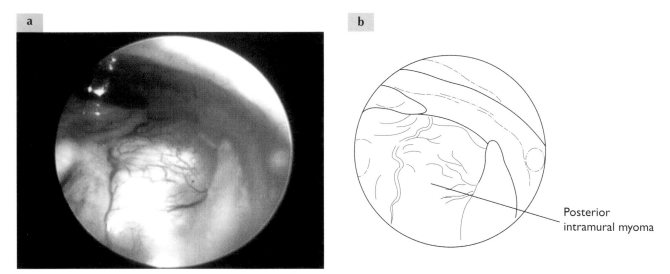

Figure 3.4 Result 7 months postoperatively: the bulge on the posterior wall of the uterus is caused by the remaining intramural portion of the myoma.

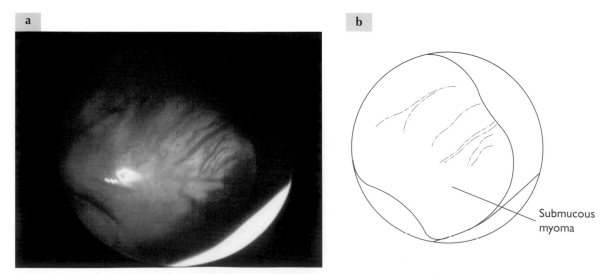

Figure 3.5 Large myoma on the right lateral wall and the posterior uterine wall of the uterus.

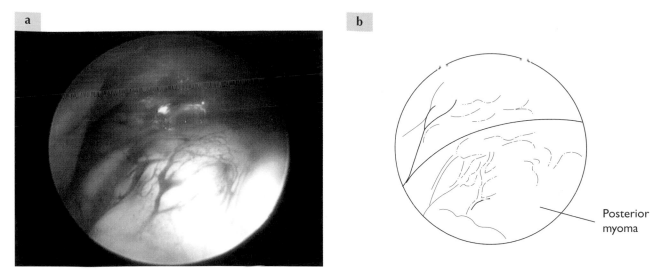

Figure 3.6 Result 1 year postoperatively: the bulge on the posterior wall is caused by secondary enucleation of the intramural portion of the myoma.

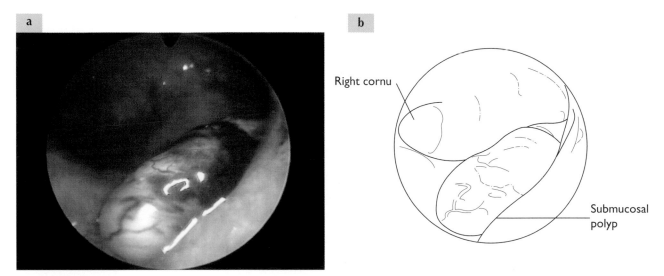

Figure 3.7 Mucosal polyp on the posterior wall.

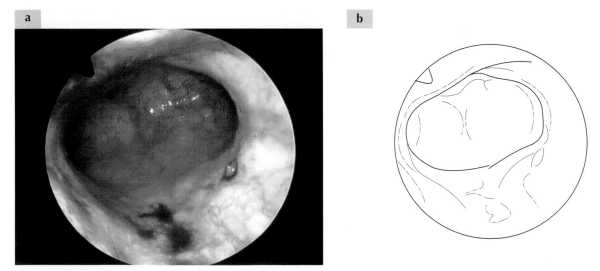

Figure 3.8 Appearance of the uterine cavity 4 months after polyp resection: excellent result.

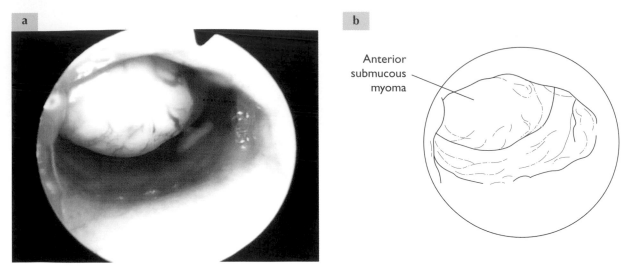

Figure 3.9 Submucosal myoma on the anterior wall.

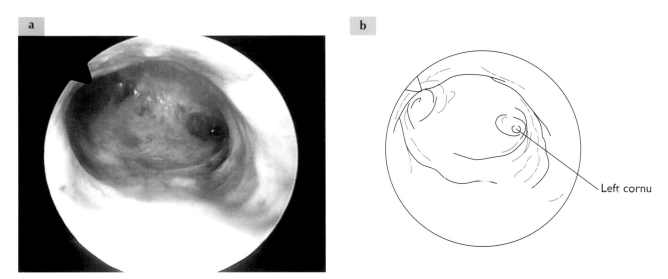

Figure 3.10 Appearance of the uterine cavity 4 months after resection: excellent result.

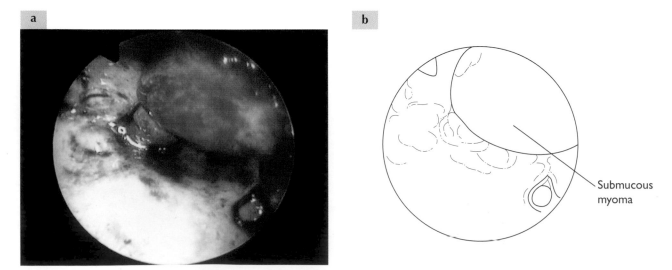

Figure 3.11 Sessile submucous myoma in the left uterine horn.

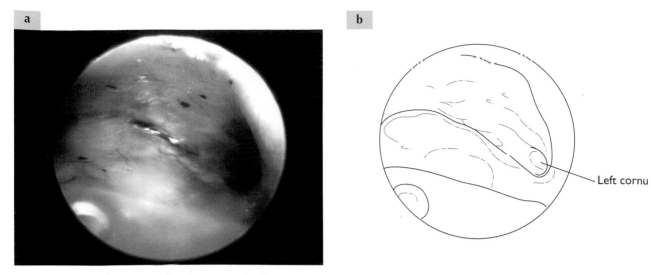

Figure 3.12 Satisfactory result seen 3 months later.

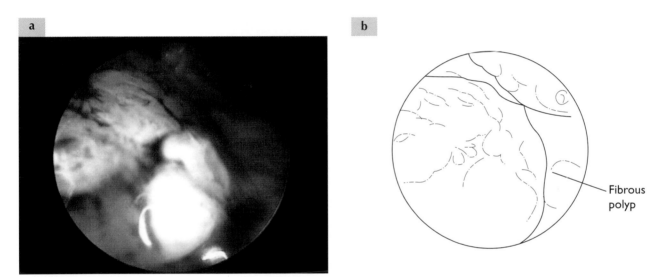

Figure 3.13 Multiple fibrous polyps on the posterior wall.

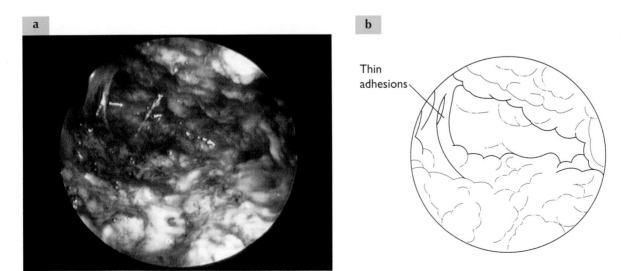

Figure 3.14 Appearance of the uterine cavity 6 months after resection of polyps and endometrial ablation by way of coagulation.

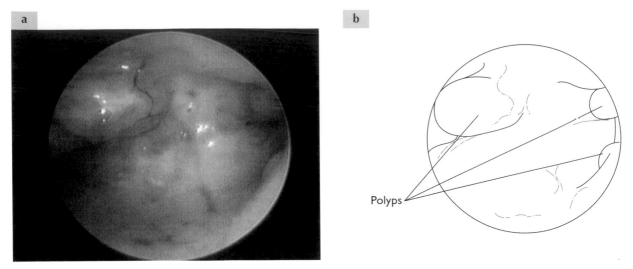

Figure 3.15 Polyp on the anterior wall of the right uterine horn and small polyps near left tubal ostium.

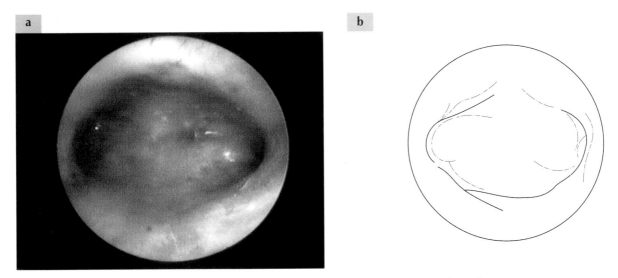

Figure 3.16 Appearance of the uterine cavity 3 months after resection: very good result.

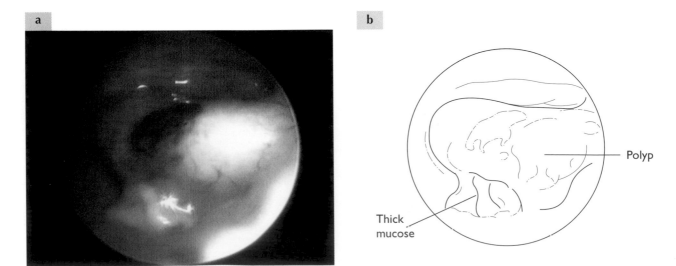

Figure 3.17 Large mucosal polyp in the left uterine horn.

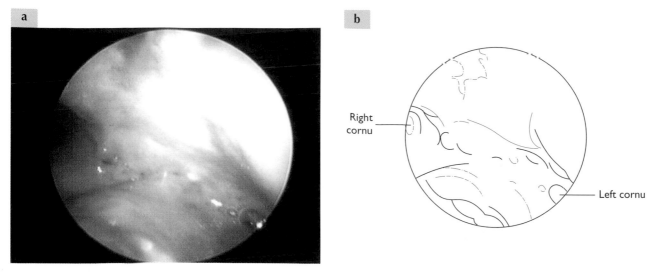

Figure 3.18 Appearance of the uterine cavity 4 months after resection: very good result.

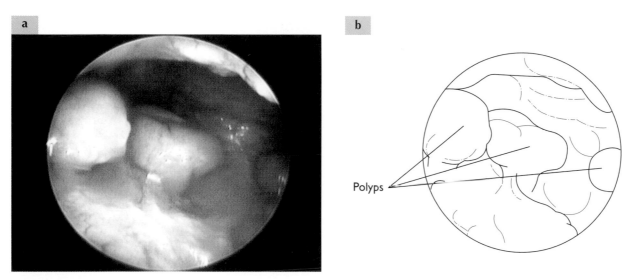

Figure 3.19 Large mucosal polyps in the uterine fundus.

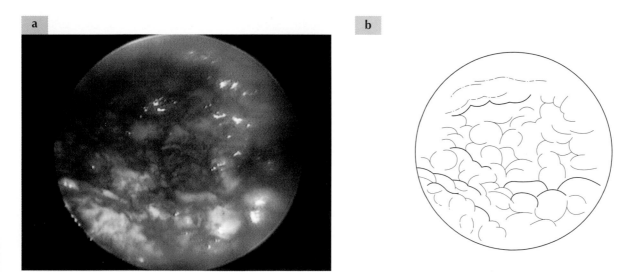

Figure 3.20 Appearance of the uterine cavity 3 months after resection of polyps and endometrial ablation: very good result.

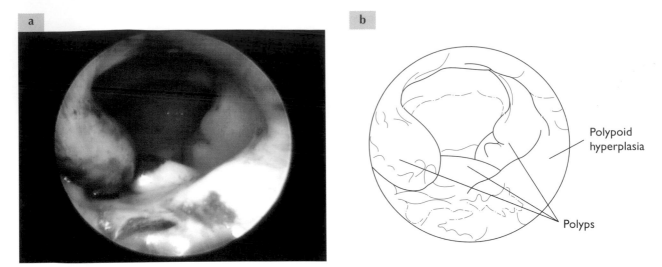

Figure 3.21 Multiple polyps and diffuse polypoid hyperplasia.

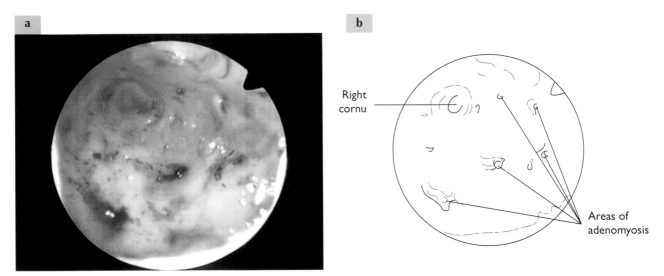

Figure 3.22 Hysteroscopic control 2 months after resection demonstrates the absence of polyps but nonetheless reveals underlying interstitial nodular adenomyosis, which was concealed by the polypoid hyperplasia.

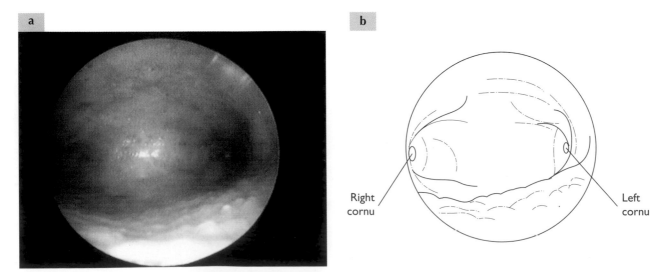

Figure 3.23 The same patient as in Fig 3.22 after 3 months of treatment with leuprolide acetate.

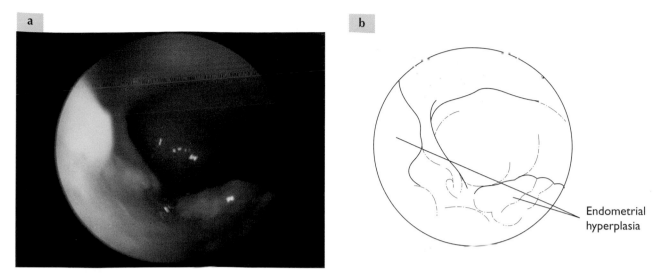

Figure 3.24 Widespread hyperplasia in the uterine cavity.

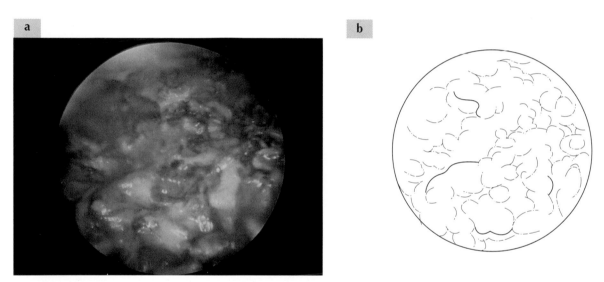

Figure 3.25 Appearance 3 months after endometrial photocoagulation ablation using Nd:YAG laser.

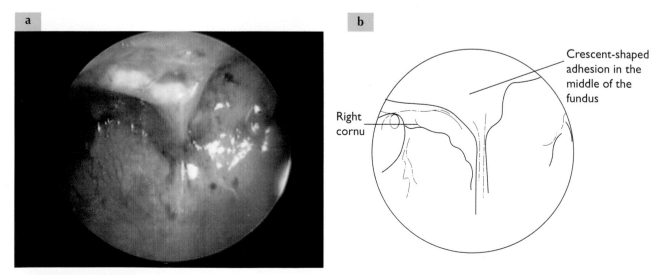

Figure 3.26 An old fibrous adhesion in the middle of the fundus.

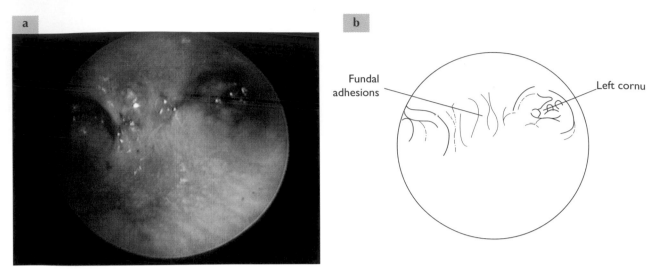

Figure 3.27 An old adhesion in the middle of the fundus (same patient as in Fig. 3.26).

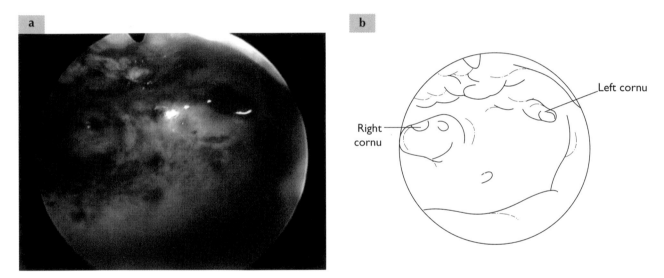

Figure 3.28 Appearance of the uterine cavity 8 months after lysis of adhesions using the Baggish hysteroscope fitted with scissors.

4 Complications

Myoma resection

Infection

Infection occurs rarely. The authors have, however, seen one case of septic necrobiosis of the residual intramural hemisphere, which required reoperation by an abdominal approach.

Bleeding

Endouterine ablation of a myoma, in the absence of perforation, usually does not cause much bleeding. As a general rule, bleeding can be controlled by selective coagulation. The placing of an indwelling catheter is an effective solution in the event of persistent postoperative bleeding. The authors have seen no cases of serious bleeding, and transfusion has not been required.

Perforation

The risk of perforation has been reported as 3–5%. The risk is greater in the case of a scarred uterus. There are two types of perforation:

- subperitoneal perforations, which are minor and are caused by false passage or a submucosal trajectory while the endocervical canal is being dilated with bougies or while the resecting instrument is being advanced; and
- intraperitoneal perforation, which can have more serious consequences; this type of perforation can be inadvertently induced at any time during the operation by a false movement of the sheath and its fittings or by an electric wire loop.

If a uterine perforation occurs, resection must be stopped, a blood assay performed, ultrasound monitoring of liquid infusion (collected in the Douglas) and antibiotics prescribed. Laparoscopy is not routinely performed, but it must be carried out if there is suspicion of damage to intra-abdominal organs. Laparoscopy is required in about one in 10 cases.

Perforation is most serious when it is directly caused by the activated wire loop. There can be a risk of profuse bleeding caused by the loss of endometrial substance due to deep ablation of the muscle. There is also a considerable risk of electrical burning if the electrode comes into contact with an abdominal organ. There have been reports of perforation of the intestinal tract during endouterine resection operations.

Endometrial ablation

Complications are rare but can be serious. A survey carried out by the American Association of Gynecologic Laparoscopists in 1988 evaluated a total risk of complications of 2% (including serious complications, at a rate of 1%). Complication rates decrease with the experience of the surgeon.

Intestinal electrical burns

The risk of intestinal electrical burns, either with or without perforation, is possible when the roller-ball electrode is used, which may cause transmural necrosis.

The prevention of this complication starts with the avoidance of false tracks, perforations and tears during the dilation of the cervix. The authors prescribe misopristol the day before the procedure to facilitate dilatation. The use of intermediate-sized Hegar bougies (number 7.5 or 8.5) is useful. Good visibility should always be preserved – the diathermy loop, roller-ball or laser fiber must remain under visual control during the operation. Detailed attention is essential at the time of the resection at the level of the uterine horns, where the subjacent myometrium is thinnest. It is preferable to extract the chips from resection progressively so as not to obstruct visibility.

Streptococcal endometritis

Postsurgical infections are rare. Their prevention rests on the injection of an intraoperative antibiotic. One case of streptococcal endometritis has been reported. It was promptly and effectively treated by antibiotics.

Pregnancy

A subsequent pregnancy may occur, if the ablation was only partial and menstrual activity continues.

Endometrial cancer discovered during histological examination of tissue removed at ablation

In a review of the literature in 1998 Valle and Baggish reported eight cases of adenocarcinoma after endometrectomy. This must encourage continuation of monitoring among women with high risk factors (e.g. diabetes, obesity, late menopause, nulliparity). Prevention requires a diagnostic hysteroscopy accompanied by an endometrial biopsy and at best by a curettage, which weighs down the procedure.

Metabolic complications arising from the distending liquid

The risk of metabolic complications arising from the distending liquid in so far as when the entire surface is affected by surgical trauma, intravasation or fluid resorption is substantially increased. Hyponatremia is a concern when excessive fluids devoid of electrolytes are absorbed (> liter).

Bleeding

Any hemorrhages are often tiny and disappear in a few hours. Prevention rests on the prevention of perforation and respect of the indications, avoiding uteri of too large a volume.

Intrauterine adhesions

There is an increased risk of perforation of the uterus in the event of complex and widespread (third-degree) adhesions. Such adhesions are dangerous because the usual landmarks (e.g. tubal openings, the uterine fundus) are obstructed. Hence, the instrument must be advanced very carefully.

The risk is increased in the case of a uterus that is fragile because of the presence of scarring or age-related atrophy, or in a uterus that is fixed in a position of retroflexion. The risk is also increased by long-standing, extensive adhesions and in patients who have been already operated on once for adhesions with unsatisfactory results.

Septum transection

One case of severe endometritis has been reported. It occurred 2 weeks after removal of a septum; an indwelling catheter also fell out. Infection with colobacilli and polymorphic flora was treated for 1 week with antibiotic infusion therapy. No perforation, bleeding or other complications occurred.

Metabolic complications

Complications involving distending liquid

Complications involving distending liquid arise from the passage of glycine into the circulatory system. The incidence varies from 0.5% to 4% depending on the series reviewed. Also referred to by urologists as the transurethral resection of the prostate syndrome (TURP), this complication is related to the mechanism of liquid reabsorption starting with transtubal passage, vascular absorption, peritoneal diffusion and particularly the dilation under pressure of the uterine vessels.

The glycine intoxication syndrome can cause:

- visual symptoms (diplopia);
- neurological symptoms (nausea, headaches, agitation, or convulsions caused by hyperammoniemic encephalopathy – the ammonia rate can reach 30–500 µmol/l);
- cardiorespiratory symptoms at a later time (pulmonary edema or collapse);
- renal failure;
- cerebral edema which can occur if more than 500 ml of glycine is absorbed; and
- hyponatremia, hypoprotinemia and a fall in hematocrit as a result of hemodilution.

These complications can be prevented through the uses of a pre-, peri-, and postoperative ionogram. Natremia, a parameter of fundamental importance, must be measured every 15 minutes. The procedure must be stopped if the serum sodium value drops below 130 mosm/l, if there are signs of fluid deficit, or if other tests and markers (e.g. pulse oximetry, esophageal temperature and urine output) show signs of decompensation.

Conclusion

The advantages of hysteroscopic surgery are numerous. It is a relatively non-invasive procedure that can be performed quickly. Furthermore, discomfort to the patient is minimal, allowing her to resume work earlier than would otherwise be the case. The major complications to be avoided are perforation of the uterus, fluid overload and acute hyponatremia caused by excessive absorption of glycine. Surgeons must be mindful of these potential complications in so far as they may be held liable for any problem arising from insufficient experience or an excessively vigorous surgical instrumentation. Surgical hysteroscopy requires perfect mastery of the diagnostic endoscope.

Bibliography

Baggish MS, Barbot J, Valle RF. *Diagnostic and operative hysteroscopy: a text and atlas.* Chicago: Year Book; 1989.

Barbot J. Nouvelles longueurs d'onde: interêt en gynécologie du laser Yag emettant à 1.32 microns. *Lett Gynecol* 1989; (suppl 112):9–10.

Bauman R, Magos AL, Kay JD, Turnbullac AC. Absorption of glycine irrigation solution during transcervical resection of endometrium. *BMJ* 1990;**300**:304–5.

Blanc B, Boubli L. Manuel d'hystéroscopie opératoire. Paris: Vigot; 1991:68–72.

Blanc B, Boubli L. Endoscopie uterine. Paris: Pradel; 1996: 117–205.

Boubli L, Blanc B, Ortage D. Complications metaboliques de l'hystéroscopie opératoire: le point de vue du chirurgien. In: *Complications de l'endoscopie operatoire en gynecologie.* Paris: Arnette; 1995:313–20.

Boubli L, Porcu G, Gandois JM, d'Ercole C, Blanc B. Risque infectieux de l'hysteroscopie. *J Gynecol Obstet Biol Reprod* 1997;**26**:250–5.

Choe JK, Baggish MS. Hysteroscopic treatment of septate uterus with neodymium Yag laser. *Fertil Steril* 1992;**57**:81–4.

Cornier E, Madelenat P, Deval B, Despierres O. Hystéroscopie diagnostique et opératoire. *Encycl Med Chir Gynecologie.* Paris: Editions Techniques; 1994;**72**:15.

Cravello L, D'Ercole C, Blanc B. Les complications des resections hystéroscopiques. *Gynecol Obstet Pratique* 1964;**84**:1–4.

Daniell JF, Bryan RK, Raymond W. Hysteroscopic endometrial ablation using the rollerball electrode. *Obstet Gynecol* 1992,**80**:329–32.

Dargent D, Mellier G, Jacquot F. Electroresection endo uterine: une serie préliminaire de 25 cas. *J Gynecol Obstet Biol Repr* 1988; **17**:940.

DeCherney A, Diamond MD, Lavy G, Polan ML. Endometrial ablation for intractable bleeding: hysteroscopic resection. *Obstet Gynecol* 1987;**70**:668–70.

DeCherney A, Polan ML. Hysteroscopic management of intrauterine lesions and intractable bleeding. *Obstet Gynecol* 1983;**61**:392–7.

Donnez J, Gillerot S, Bougonjon D *et al.* Neodymium:YAG laser hysteroscopy in large submucous fibroids. *Fertil Steril* 1990;**54**:999–1003.

Dubuisson JB, Morice P, Chapron C. Traitement endoscopique des myomes uterins. *Ref Gynecol Obstet* 1995;**4**:387–95.

Gervaise A, Fernandez H, Capella-Allone S *et al.* Thermal balloon ablation versus endometrial resection for the treatment of abnormal uterine bleeding. *Hum Reprod* 1999;**14**:2743–7.

Gimpelson RJ. Hysteroscopic NdYAG laser ablation of the endometrium. *J Reprod Med* 1988;**33**:872–6.

Golfier F, Raudrant. La resection endometriale hystéroscopique: une alternative à l'hystérectomie. *Forum Gynecol* 1996;**5**:2–3.

Guedj H. Videohysteroscopie: diagnostics. Presénce et communications médicales (Laboratoires Wyeth France). *Gynform* 1995;**6**:9–12.

Guedj H, Valle RF. A slide atlas of hysteroscopy: an aid to diagnosis. Carnforth: Parthenon; 1995.

Guedj H, Valle RF. An atlas of hysteroscopy: a guide to diagnosis. The Encyclopedia of Visual Medicine Series. Carnforth: Parthenon; 1997.

Hallez JP. Single stage total hysteroscopic myomectomies: indications, techniques and results. *Fertil Steril* 1995;**63**:703–8.

Hallez JP, Netter A, Cartier R. Methodical intrauterine resection. *Am J Obstet Gynecol* 1987;**156**:1080–4.

Hill D, Maher P, Wood C, Lawrence A, Downing B, Lolatgis N. Complications of operative hysteroscopy. *Gynaecol Endosc* 1992;**1**:185–9.

Istre O, Bjoennes J, Naess R, Hornbaek K, Forman A. Post operative cerebral oedema after transcervical endometrial resection and uterine irrigation with 1.5% glycine. *Lancet* 1994;**344**:1187–9.

Jourdain O, Descamps P, Alle C *et al.* Traitement des fibromes. *Ref Gynecol Obstet* 1993;**6**:520–6.

Lin BL, Niyamoto N, Aoki R, Iwata Y, Irzuka R. Transcervical resection of submucous myoma. *Nippon Sanka Fujinka Gakkai Zassh*, 1986;**38**:1647–52.

Loffer FD. Removal of large symptomatic intrauterine growths by the hysteroscopic resectoscope. *Obstet Gynecol* 1990;**76**:836–40.

Neuwirth RS. Hysteroscopic management of symptomatic submucous fibroids. *Obstet Gynecol* 1983;**62**:509–11.

Neuwirth RS, Amin HK. Excision of submucous fibroids with hysteroscopic control. *Am J Obstet Gynecol* 1976;**126**:95–9.

Neuwirth RS, Dura AS, Singer A et al. The endometrial ablator: a new instrument. *Obstet Gynecol* 1994;**83**:792–6.

Magos A, Bauman R, Turnbull A. Transcervical resection of endometrium in women with metrorrhagia. *BMJ*, 1989;**298**:1209–12.

Paces S, Labri F, Lotti G. LH-RH analogues in the preparation of uterine fibromyoma. *Minerva Gynecol* 1992;**44**:245–50.

Parent B, Barbot J, Guedj H, Nodarian P. Hystéroscopie chirurgicale: laser et techniques classiques. 2nd ed. Paris: Masson; 1997:65–116.

Parent B, De Cuypere F. Traitement des fibromes uterins par hystéroscopie chirurgicale. *Abstr Gynecol* 1996;**158**:12–13.

Parent B, Guedj H. Ce qu'il faut expliquer à une femme qui va se faire opérer d'un fibrome sous hystéroscopie. *Quotidien Med* 1994;**5404**:16–17.

Rock JA, Jones HW Jr. The clinical management of tho double uterus. *Fertil Steril* 1977;**28**:798–806.

Siegler AM, Valle RF. Therapeutic hysteroscopic procedures. *Fertil Steril* 1988;**50**:685–701.

Siegler AM, Valle RF, Lindemann HJ, Mencaglia L. *Therapeutic hysteroscopy. Indications and techniques.* St. Louis: Mosby; 1990.

Valle RF. Hysteroscopic treatment of partial and complete uterine septum. *Int J Fertil* 1996;**41**:310–15.

Valle RF. Operative hysteroscopy and resectoscopy. In: Sanfilippo JS, Levine RL, eds. *Operative gynecologic endoscopy*. New York: Springer; 1996:315–47.

Valle RF, Baggish MS. Endometrial carcinoma after endometrial ablation: high-risk factors predicting its occurrence. *Am J Obstet Gynecol* 1998;**179**:569–72.

Valle RF, Sciarra JJ. Intrauterine adhesions: hysteroscopic diagnosis, classification, treatment, and reproductive outcome. *Am J Obstet Gynecol* 1988;**158**:1459–70.

Appendix: pathology and diagnosis

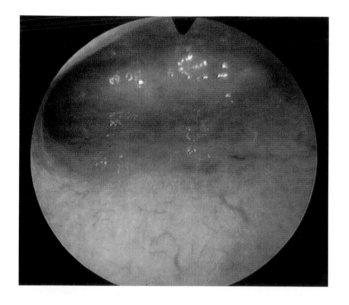

Normal uterine visualization

Figure A1 Normal uterine cavity in the postmenstrual phase (day 5 or 6): the endometrium immediately after menstruation is thin, yellowish red, and the denuded surface is fairly smooth, showing the remnants of eroded glands.

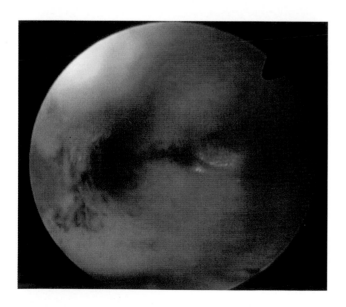

Figure A2 Normal uterine cavity in the regenerative phase (days 7 to 10), also called the preovulatory stage: the endometrium is thinnest and looks velvety. This is the best period in which to perform hysteroscopy.

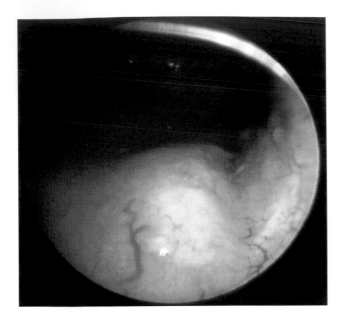

Figure A3 Normal uterine cavity in the secretory phase (days 15 to 26) or luteal stage: edematous stroma with imprint of the endoscope left on the mucosa is indicative of active growth of the endometrium. The glands become wavy, tortuous and swollen; many dented ostia are scattered on the surface.

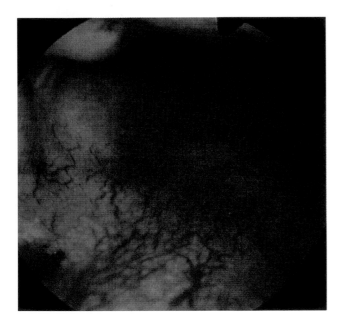

Figure A4 Normal uterine cavity in the premenstrual phase (days 27 and 28): the endometrium during the involution phase presents a wrinkled surface, and subepithelial blood vessels are visible (groups of coiled arteries).

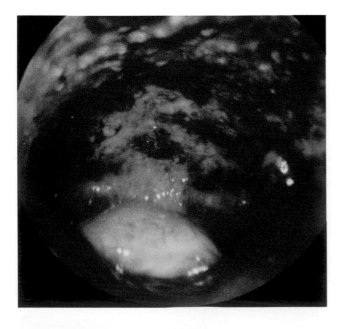

Figure A5 Uterine cavity in the menstrual phase with a polyp on the posterior wall: the desquamation of the endometrium is almost completed; on the third day of menstruation, the surface is covered with several tiny projections of stumps of glands and blood vessels.

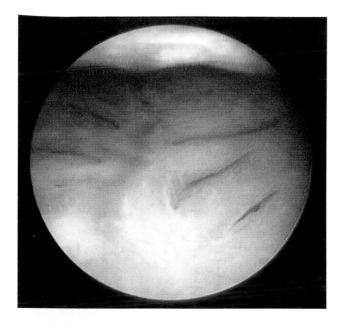

Figure A6 Endocervical canal in the nulliparous woman: the canal of the cervix is spindle-shaped, the mucosa projects into the canal and fans out as the longitudinal crests and plicae palmatae with secondary oblique branching give the appearance of a tree ("arbor vitae"). The color is light pink.

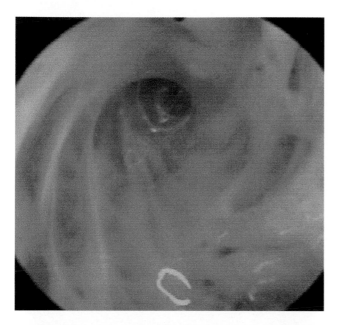

Figure A7 Endocervical canal in the multiparous woman: the mucosa shows numerous folds and clefts, aspect depending on individual variation and parity.

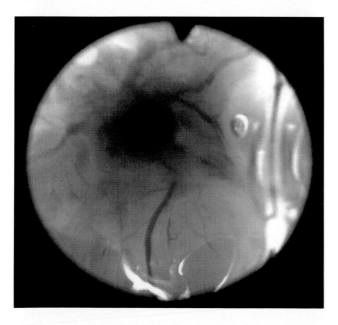

Figure A8 Internal os beginning to open: during this phase of examination, with low pressure-CO_2, hysteroscopy shows a pink mucosa with many fine, branched vessels.

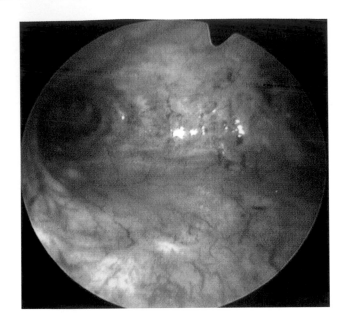

Figure A9 Uterine cavity in postmenopausal woman: the endometrium shows extensive atrophy; the courses of small blood vessel are clearly discernible, which accounts for abnormal bleeding.

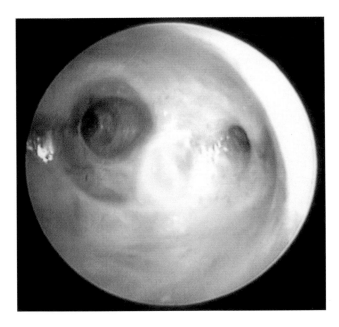

Figure A10 Uterine cavity in senile woman: the surface of the atrophic endometrium is completely flat. The mucosa, now thin, bright and glossy, has lost all relief. Vascularization becomes scarce. The two tubal ostia are clearly visible. The muscle fibers are ivory-white in color. No bleeding can occur.

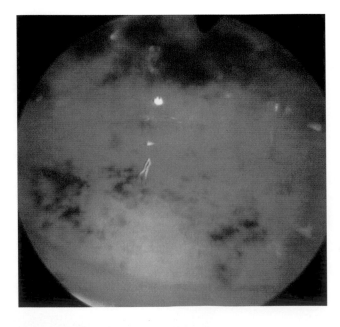

Endometrium treated by birth control pills

Figure A11 Uterine cavity in woman taking oral contraceptives: the endometrium is more often sub-atrophic with subepithelial blood vessels and small hematomas visible though the stroma. The occurrence of breakthrough bleeding is not uncommon.

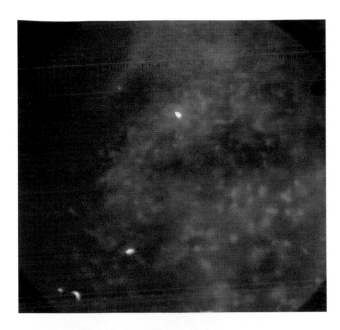

Endometritis

Figure A12 Hysteroscopic view of chronic endometritis: the endometrium is finely wrinkled all over, with areas of epithelium a reddish brown in color, and scattered bright points (strawberry aspect). Chronic endometritis may also be associated with tumors (leiomyoma, endometrial polyp or endometrial cancer) or retained gestational tissue or an IUD.

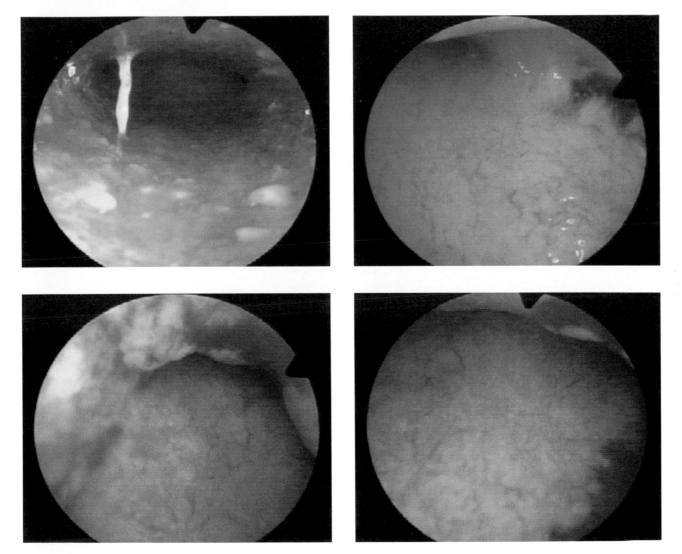

Figure A13 Hysteroscopic findings of acute endometritis: a fine network of subepithelial blood vessels spreading all over the surface epithelium. An edematous endometrium, with areas of bleeding occasionally associated with many small elevations evoking micro polyps, can also be seen. The assessment of this endometrium was performed as part of an infertility examination before a hysteroscopic transfer (in vitro fertilization IVF) in a woman who had undergone many treatments without success.

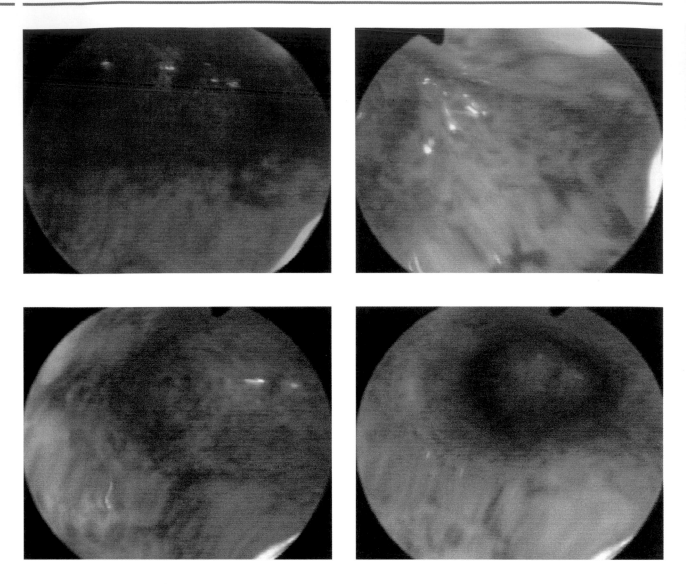

Uterine anomalies

Figure A14 Hysteroscopic assessment in a DES-exposed girl: displaying a cylindrical shaped and hypoplastic cavity with shallow cornua, the two ostia are well visible.

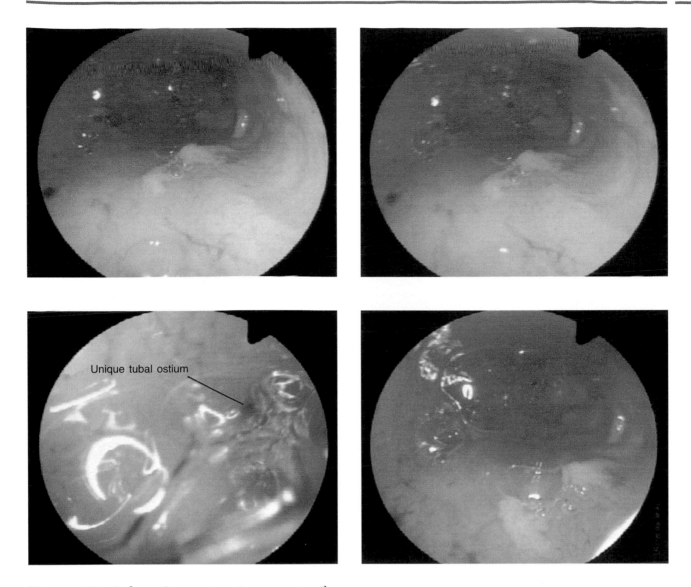

Figure A15 Left unicornuate uterus: note the narrowness of the semi cavity and the unique tubal ostium on the left.

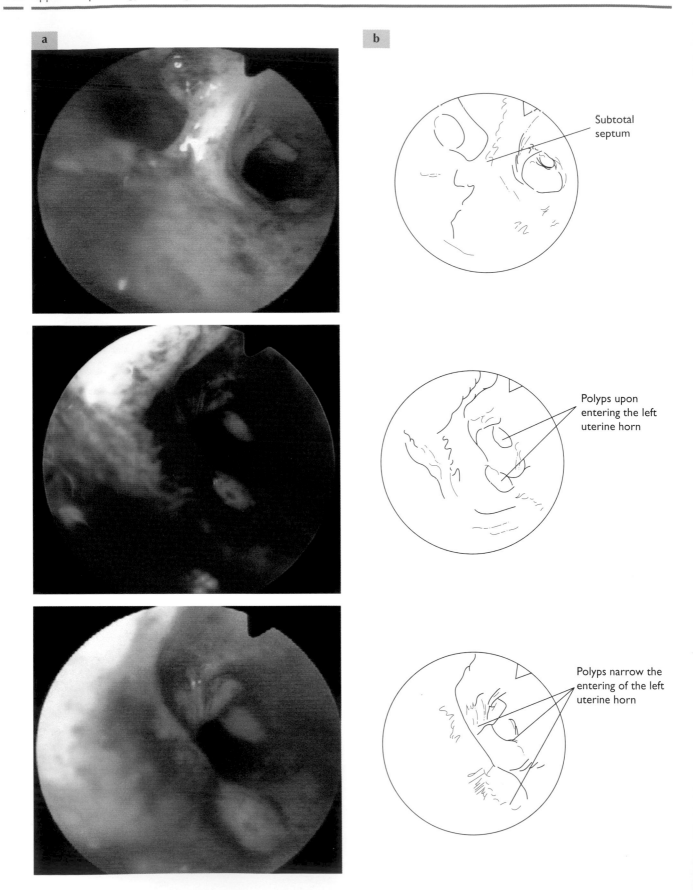

Figure A16 Septate uterus. Only the septate uterus is amenable to hysteroscopic metroplasty.

a,b Subtotal septate uterus and polyps: the lower extremity of the septum is at the level of the isthmus. A full panorama with the tubal orifices in plain sight appears immediately upon entering the cavity. A close-up view of left uterine cornu shows two small polyps on the anterior wall and the posterior wall.

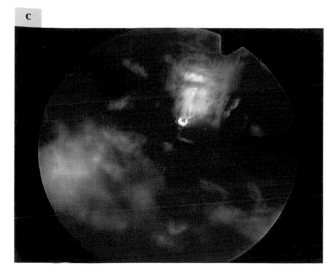

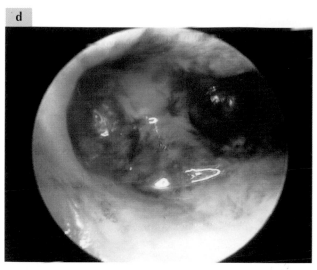

c Corporeal septate or partial septate uterus: the broad septum occupies only the third superior part of the uterine cavity separating two uterine horns and extends about 3 cm into uterine cavity.

d Arcuate or 'cordiform uterus' is a minor uterine malformation caused by failure of complete fusion of Müllerian ducts; a fundal indentation separates the two tubal orifices. On hysterography, the contour is that of a saddle-shaped fundus. This type of uterine anomaly is considered a normal variant and is not associated with infertility or obstetrical difficulties.

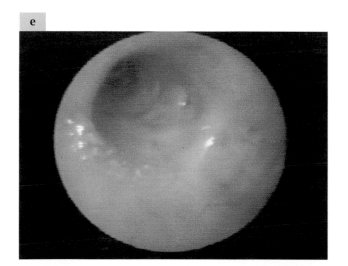

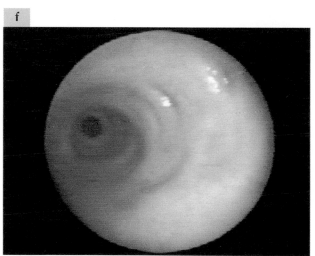

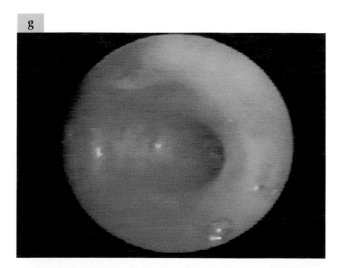

Bicornuate uterus: partial bicornuate variety; visualization of the cornua requires that the hysteroscope be advanced further because of the angle between the isthmus and the uterine corpus, the two tubal orifices cannot appear in plain sight.

e Isthmus.
f Right uterine horn.
g Left uterine horn.

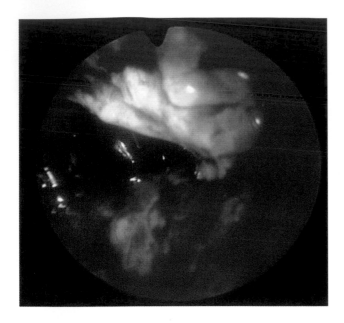

Endometrial hyperplasia

Figure A17 Localized hyperplasia on the anterior wall and the left edge of the isthmus.

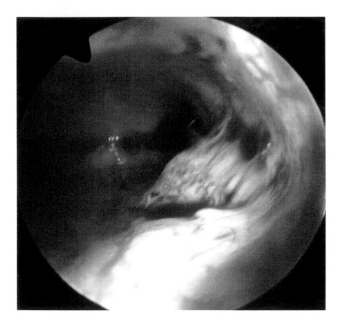

Figure A18 Localized hyperplasia on the left side of the left uterine horn.

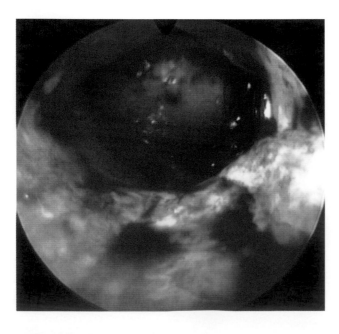

Figure A19 Localized hyperplasia on the posterior wall of the uterine cavity.

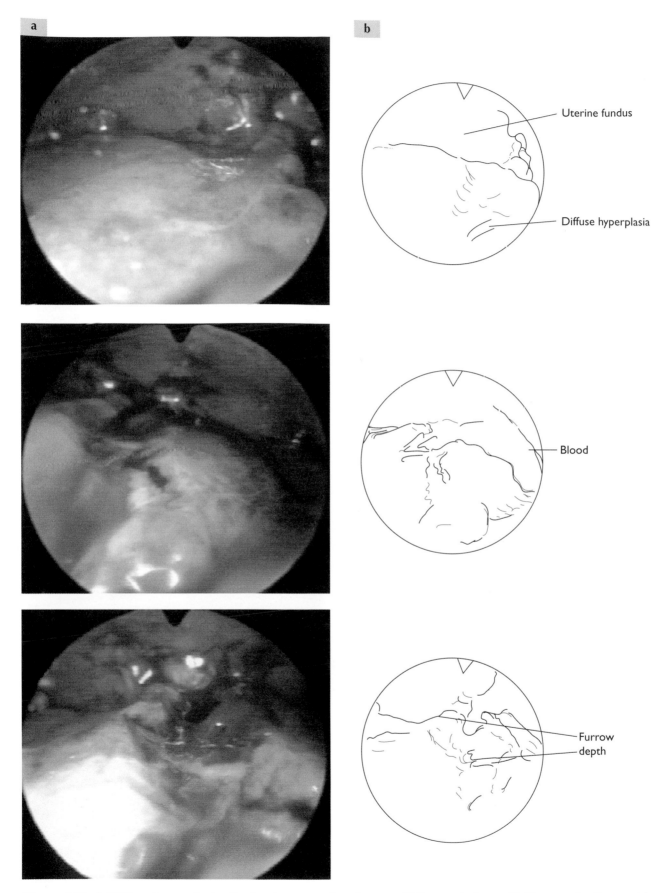

Figure A20a,b Diffuse hyperplasia: the hysteroscope has "grooved" the posterior wall. Furrow depth provides an indication of the thickness of the uterine mucosa. After curettage, the histological examination showed a polypoid hyperplasia.

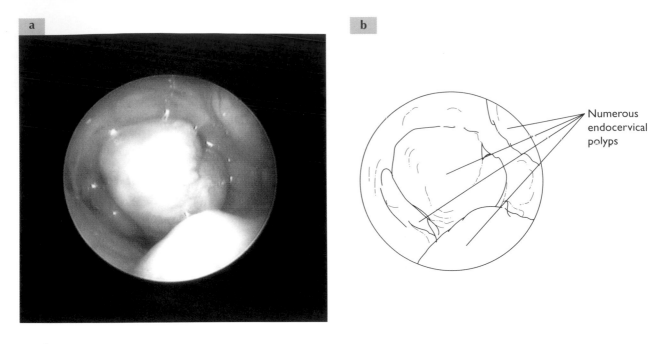

Polyps

Figure A21a,b Numerous polyps filling the endo-cervical canal.

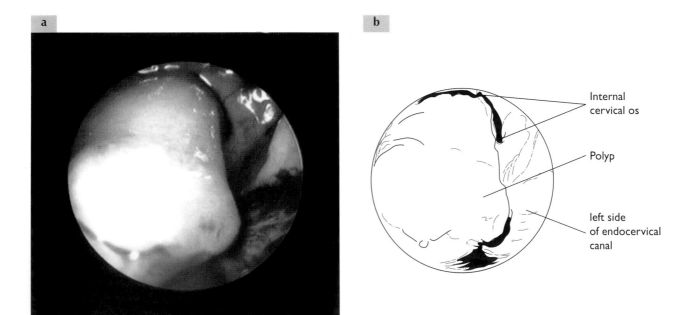

Figure A22a,b Large mucous polyp protruding through the internal cervical os into the endocervical canal.

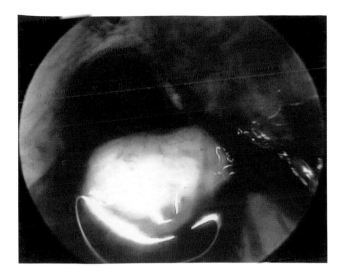

Figure A23 Large sessile polyp on the posterior wall of the endocervical canal.

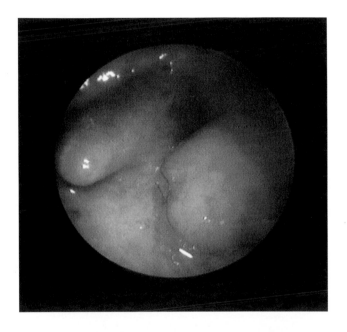

Figure A24 Broad-based pedicles of two polyps on the uterine fundus.

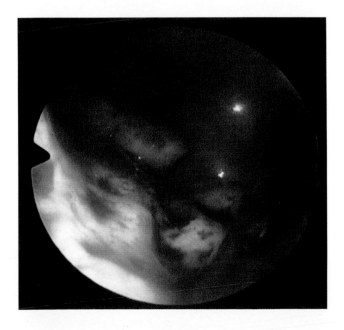

Figure A25 Multiple polyps on the posterior wall of the uterus.

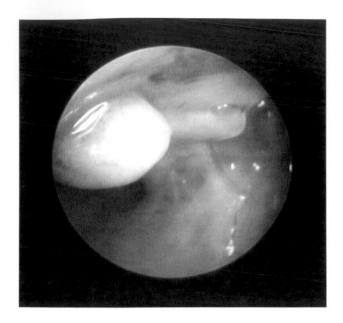

Figure A26 Sessile polyps located on the anterior wall of the right uterine horn.

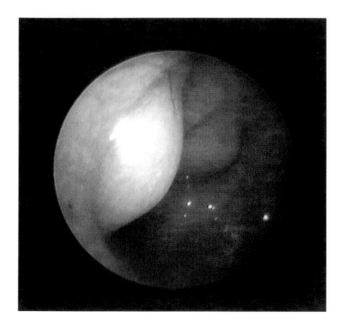

Figure A27 Functional polyps covered with normal endometrium huddled in the right uterine horn. The tubal ostium is just behind the polyp.

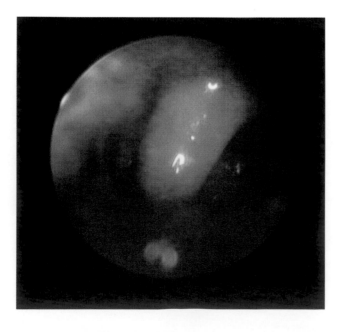

Figure A28 Functional linguiform polyp arising from the uterine fundus, reminiscent of the palative ovula.

a

b

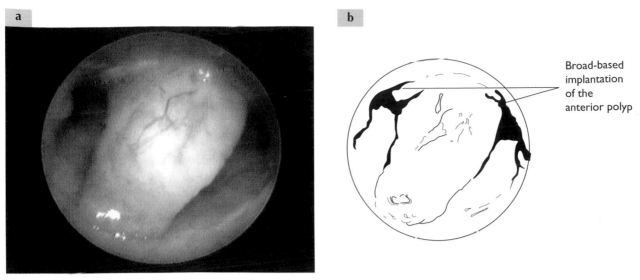

Figure A29 Pedunculated polyp arising from the anterior uterine wall.

a

b

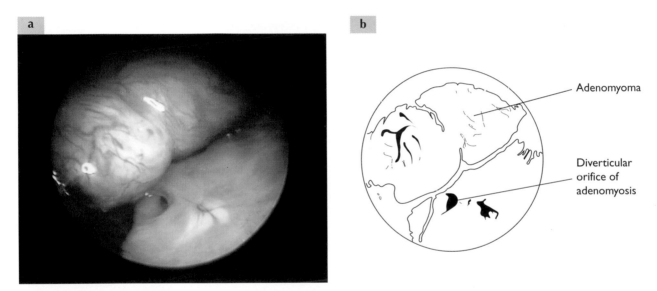

Figure A30a,b Endometrial polyp lying on the posterior uterine wall, that was diagnosed as an adenomyoma on histologic examination. Note the diverticular orifice of adenomyosis just below.

a

b

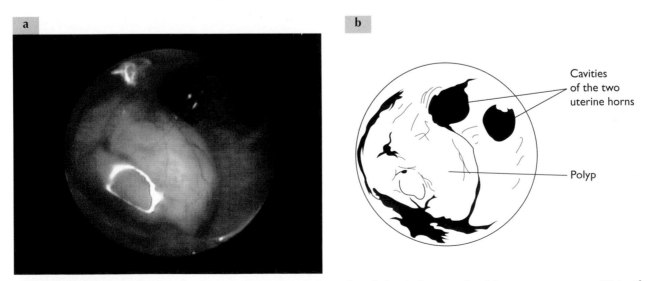

Figure A31a,b Spherical polyp located on the right side of the isthmus of a bicornuate uterus. Note the cavities of the two uterine horns just above.

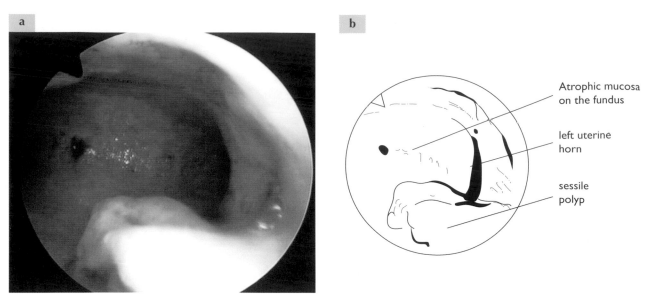

Figure A32a,b Sessile non-functional polyp on the posterior uterine wall: note that the color of the polyp is not the same as that of the surrounding endometrium.

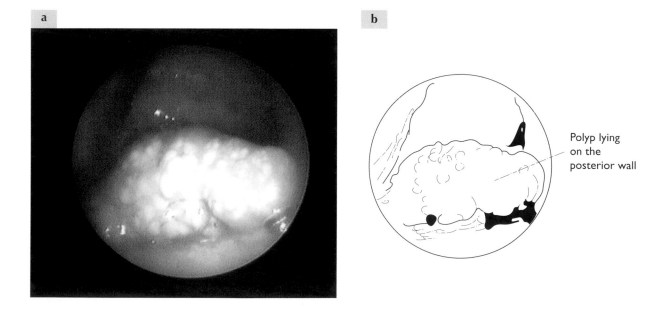

Misleading hysteroscopic images

Figure A33a,b Difficult hysteroscopic assessment of a polypoid image: histological examination diagnosed a fibroid polyp with dystrophic endometrium and small cystic glandular structures typical of polypoid hyperplasia, without signs of high-risk endometrial hyperplasia.

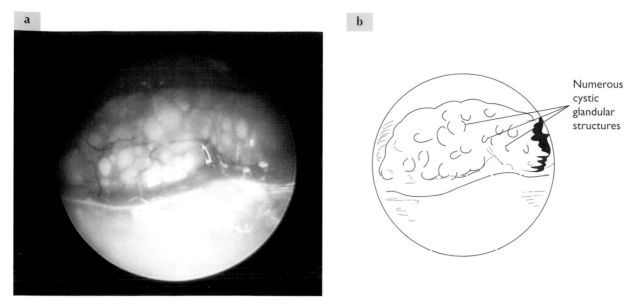

Figure A34a,b Close-up view of the dystrophic endometrial polyp: note the numerous small cysts on the surface of the polyp.

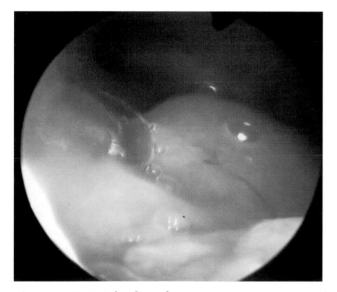

Figure A35 Misleading hysteroscopic images: on histologic examination this polypoid hyperplasia was in fact a leiomyoma.

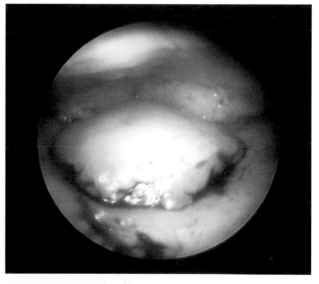

Figure A36 Misleading hysteroscopic images: the bizarre configuration of this lesion evoked a polyp or a polypoid form of cancer, or an endometrial ossification. Histological examination after resection showed a simple mucous polyp.

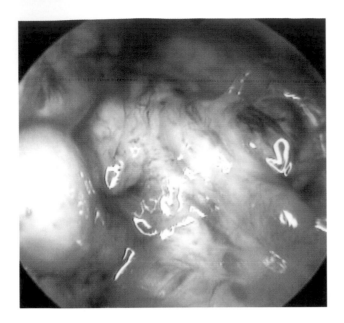

Figure A37 Misleading hysteroscopic images: close-up view of this lesion showing atypical hyperplasia, where superficial capillary vascularization takes on a bizarre configuration exhibiting a "corkscrew" pattern. After resection, histological examination revealed mucous fibroid polyps.

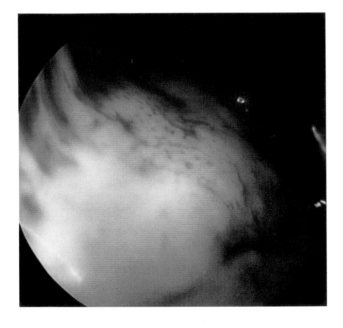

Fibromas

Figure A38 Submucous fibroma involving the entire posterior uterine wall, largely intramural, during an episode of bleeding. Blood oozes from the network of dilated vessels.

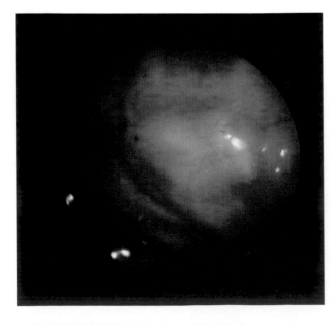

Figure A39 Enormous fibroma bulging into the uterine cavity: hysteroscopic removal is more difficult, the risks of perforation and metabolic complications are greater. However, use of the resectoscope combined with laser and ultrasound monitoring of the procedure allows safe resection of the myoma.

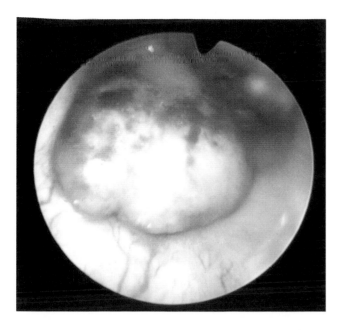

Figure A40 Voluminous pedunculated endometrial polyp: broad-based pedicle arising from the anterior uterine wall. Histological examination resulted in accurate diagnosis of fibro-mucous and glandular cystic polyp.

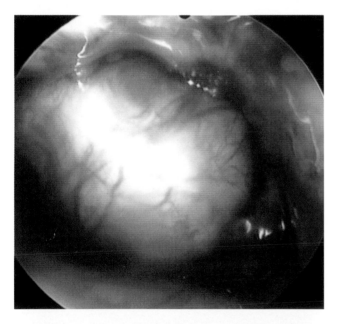

Figure A41 A broad-based pedunculated myoma implanted on the anterior wall.

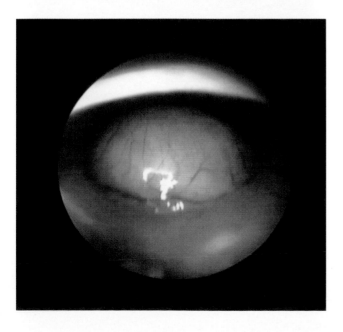

Figure A42 Sessile semispherical fibroma on the posterior wall.

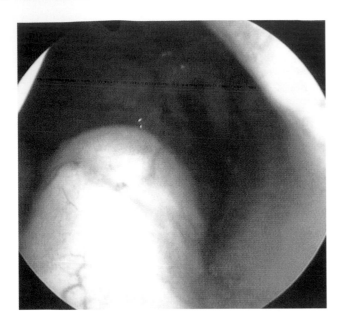

Figure A43 Hysteroscopic view of an intramural and submucous myoma arising from the posterior wall of the uterus and pressing inward to deform and constrict the uterine cavity.

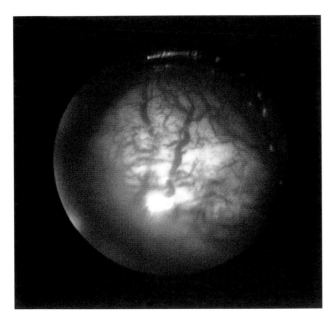

Figure A44 Submucosal myoma with extensive vascular pattern.

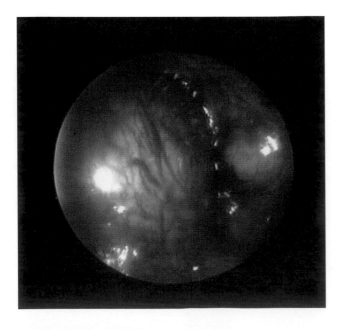

Figure A45 Same fibroma Figure A44: exploration of the uterine cavity shows that two submucous myomas are juxtaposed.

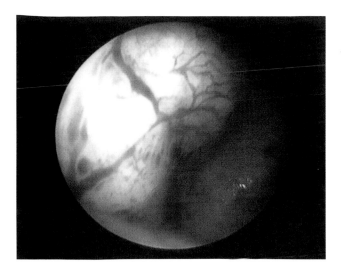

Figure A46 Submucous myoma deforming the right side of the uterine cavity: numerous thin-walled sinusoidal vessels are seen coursing over the white myoma.

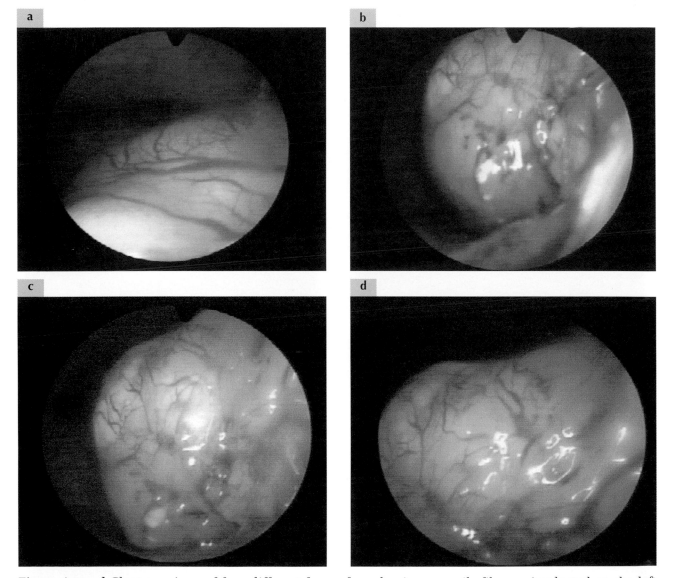

Figure A47a–d Close-up views of four different faces of a voluminous sessile fibroma implanted on the left side of the uterine cavity: note the surface vessels and its projection into the uterine cavity.

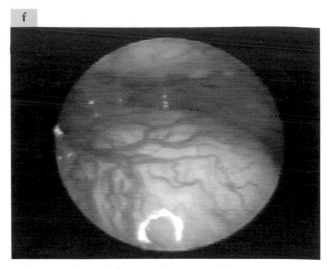

Figure A47e,f Submucous myoma protruding into the uterine cavity, with extensive vascular pattern.

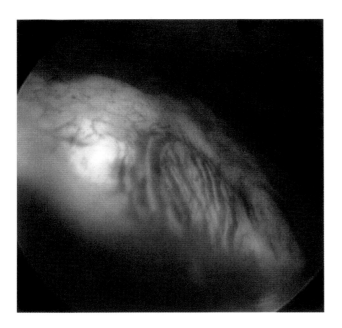

Figure A48 Submucosal myoma of the posterior wall: this tumor represents only a small portion protruding into the uterine cavity; most of the myoma is largely intramural.

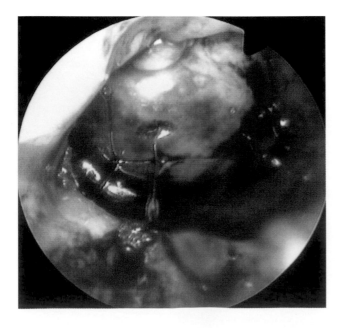

Figure A49 Sessile submucous myoma on the anterior uterine wall.

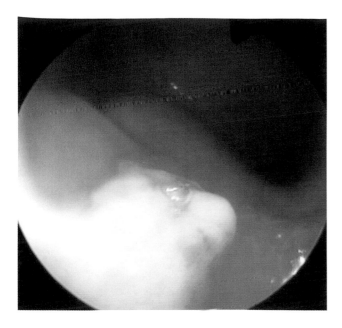

Figure A50 Hysteroscopic view of multiple myomas on the posterior wall, masked by a diffuse endometrial hyperplasia.

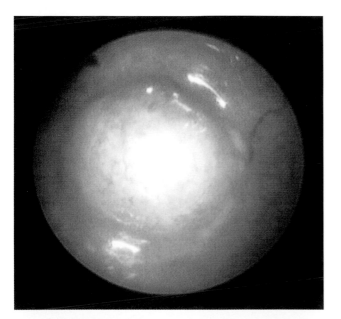

Figure A51 Semispherical fibroma occupying the uterine fundus.

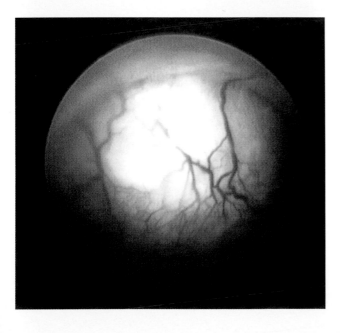

Figure A52 Typical submucous myoma with vascular pattern somewhat inhibited by preadministration of GnRH agonists.

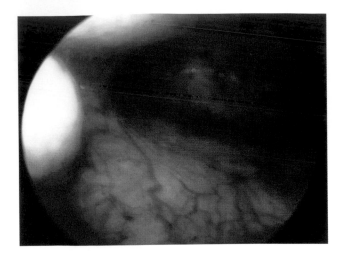

Figure A53 Small sessile fibroma of the right side of the uterine cavity: the endometrium overlaying the myoma can be examined with its vascular pattern.

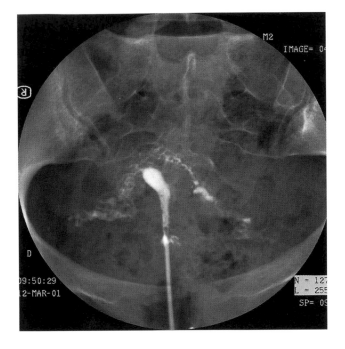

Intrauterine adhesions

Figure A54 Hysterography suggestive of a unicornuate uterus. In fact, hysteroscopy revealed the presence of large uterine adhesion obliterating the left uterine horn. This woman had undergone a curettage after a delivery 10 years before and had an amenorrhea 6 months previously. The endometrium seems more vulnerable to injury during the early postpartum phase.

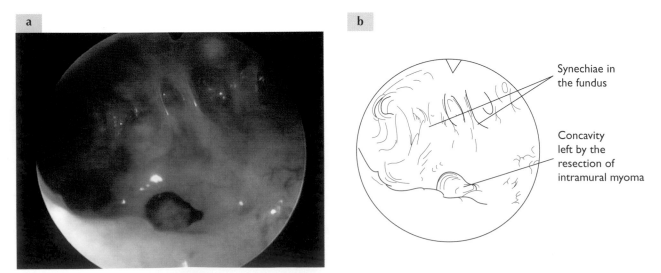

Figure A55a,b Intrauterine adhesion of the uterine fundus following the resection of multiple submucous myomas. Note on the posterior wall the concavity left by the resection of the intraparietal portion of one of the myomas.

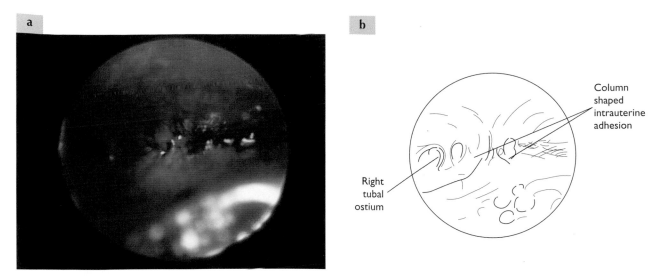

Figure A56a,b Intrauterine adhesion of the uterine fundus following curettage for evacuation of an incomplete spontaneous abortion (about one-third of intrauterine adhesions).

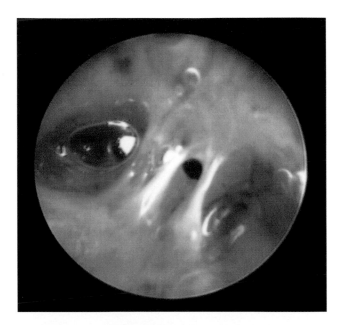

Figure A57 Intrauterine adhesion of the isthmus: the internal cervical os is either invisible or opens onto a short, funnel-shaped cavity.

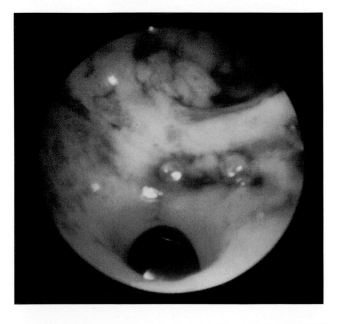

Figure A58 A large corporeal intrauterine adhesion: in this case, the extensive adhesion is made up entirely of connective tissue. The epithelial cover is flat and atrophic, white, and only marginally vascularized. The surface has a bright appearance.

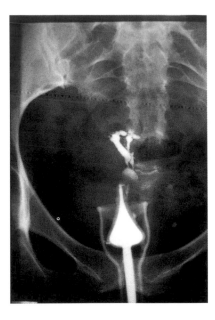

Figure A59 Radiological image of the same intrauterine adhesion as Fig. A58.

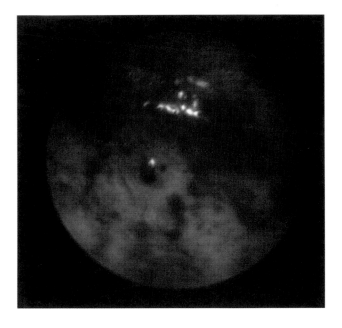

Adenomyosis

Figure A60 Diverticular adenomyosis on the posterior wall near the fundus: on hysteroscopy it appears in the form of a small brownish spot which is a small depression within the mucosa. Note the hypervascularization of the endometrium, which is fragile.

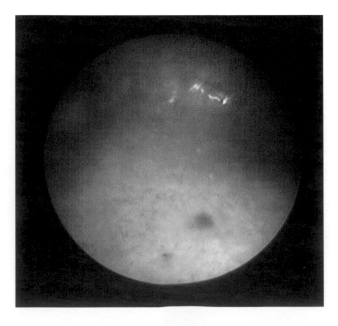

Figure A61 Interstitial adenomyosis on the posterior uterine wall: it actually corresponds to islands of adenomyosis that have lost their direct connection with the surface of endometrium.

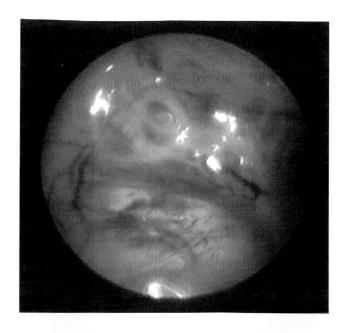

Figure A62 Brownish diverticula and myometrial hypertrophy are visible in the fundus, numerous thin-walled sinusoidal vessels are seen coursing over the endometrium of the posterior wall: they are signs of adenomyosis.

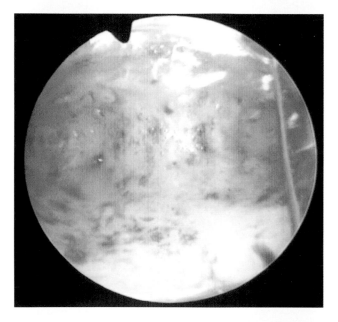

Figure A63 Diffuse interstitial adenomyosis: result after 3 months of administration of GnRH analogs: the treatment has atrophied the uterine mucosa, the increased vascularization is no longer visible, and some islands of adenomyosis are still visible.

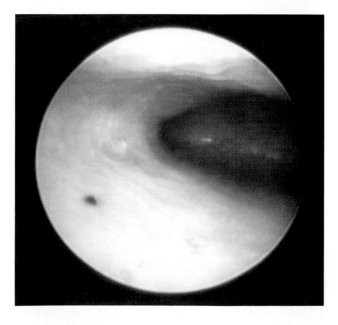

Figure A64 Focal interstitial adenomyosis: the brownish focus of adenomyosis is visible on the posterior wall near the right uterine side.

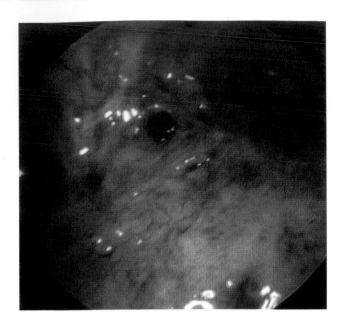

Figure A65–67 Three steps in the treatment of an important diverticular adenomyosis with GnRH analogs.

Figure A65 Close-up of the uterine fundus showing diverticula and trabeculate appearance resulting from hypertrophic muscular columns. The endometrial surface is hemorrhagic.

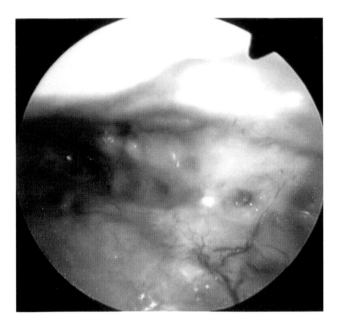

Figure A66 The same patient after ovarian suppression with gonadotropin-releasing hormone agonists over 3 months: atrophy of endometrium, diverticula and vessels are shown.

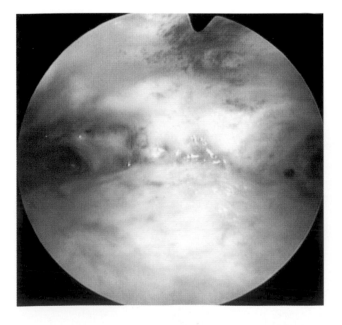

Figure A67 The same patient after 6 months of treatment with GnRH analogs: the treatment atrophies the uterine mucosa to the extent that it disappears. However, the medical treatment of adenomyosis only provides a transitory break in the progress of the disease.

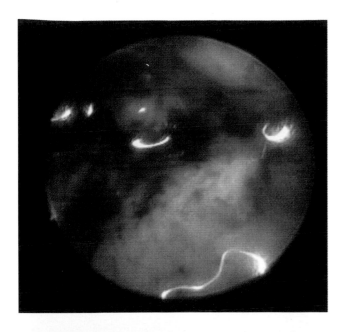

Endometrial carcinoma

Figure A68 Endometrial carcinoma: this well-differentiated adenocarcinoma is a purely mucosal cancer; surface extension with cobblestone appearance, conspicuous and uneven vascularization.

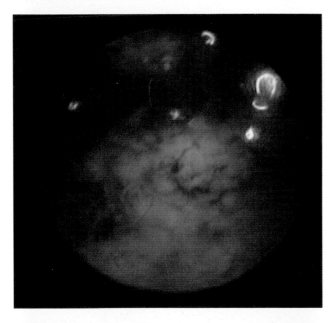

Figure A69 Close-up view of the same adenocarcinoma: if the endoscope is brought up against the tumor, the vascularization can be easily seen: blood vessels are numerous, distended and meandering, sometimes with thrombosis.

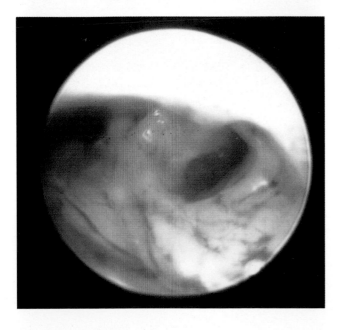

Figure A70 Endometrial adenocarcinoma moderately differentiated: the tumor consists of many large buds which occupy the high part of the uterus and penetrate the right uterine horn.

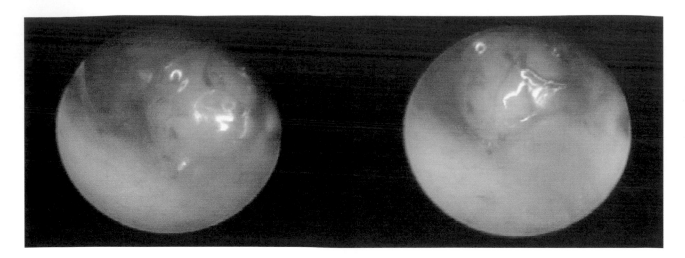

Tamoxifen effects

Figure A71 Tamoxifen has been implicated in an increased rate of hyperplasia, endometrial polyps and perhaps endometrial carcinoma. Here, an endometrial polyp in a woman who had received tamoxifen treatment for breast cancer for 3 years; histologic examination diagnosed an endometrial mucous polyp, with glandular cystic areas.

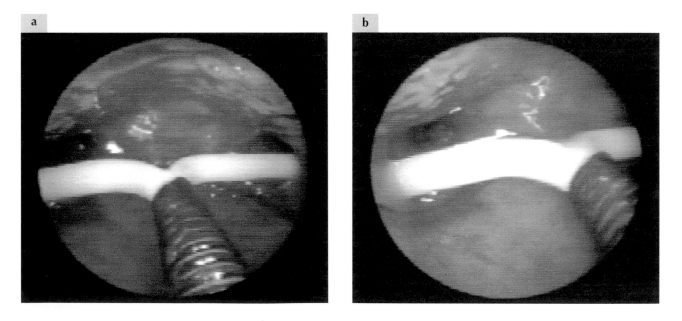

IUDs

Figure A72 T-shaped device (Nova T) associated with chronic endometritis: tiny whitish papillary projections are due to local responses of the endometrium to chronic inflammation (a). Note the right arm of the IUD is covered with a coating of pus (b). The IUD was used for 7 years; the patient developed prolonged menstrual flow, temporary spotting and menstrual colic.

Operative hysteroscopic views

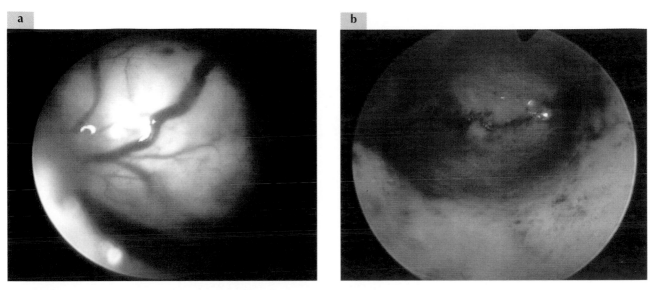

Figure A73 (a) A broad-based pedunculated myoma located on the right lateral wall of the uterus. (b) appearance of the uterine cavity 2 months after resection.

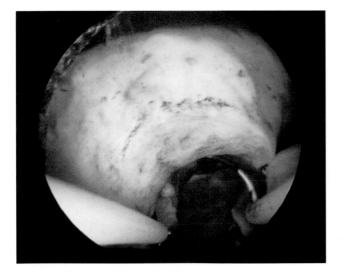

Figure A74 Resection of a myoma of the anterior wall. The resectoscopic cutting loop is placed behind the myoma and is engaged. The power is turned on and the loop is drawn back toward the hysteroscopic sheath. The resection is not hemorrhagic.

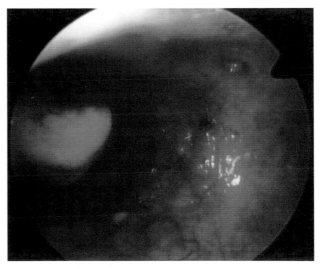

Figure A75 Old placental polyp found in the right uterine horn 1 year after an abortion.

Index